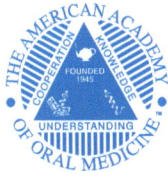

CLINICIAN'S GUIDE
Treatment of Patients with HIV & Other Communicable Diseases
FIFTH EDITION

EDITORS

Brian C. Muzyka, DMD, MS, MBA
Associate Professor
Director Hospital Dentistry
Vidant Medical Center
East Carolina University
School of Dental Medicine
Greenville, North Carolina

CONTRIBUTING AUTHORS

Kimberly R. Dehler, MS, DDS
Rodolfo N. Epifanio, DDS
Dena J. Fischer, DDS, MSD, MS
Jananya Plianrungsi, DDS
Caroline H. Shiboski, DDS, MPH, PhD
Juan F. Yepes, DDS, MD, MPH, MS, DrPH

PREVIOUS EDITION CONTRIBUTORS

Lauren L. Patton, DDS
Joel B. Epstein, DMD, MSD
Stephen N. Abel, DDS, MS
Michael Glick, DMD

The authors are members of the American Academy of Oral Medicine. This monograph represents a consensus of the contributing authors and not necessarily the private views of any of the individuals

CONTENTS

American Academy of Oral Medicine
2150 N. 107th St., Suite 205
Seattle, Washington 98133
TEL: (206) 209-5279
EMAIL: info@aaom.com   WEBSITE: www.aaom.com
©2018 American Academy of Oral Medicine

ISBN
Paperback: 978-1-936176-53-3
PDF: 978-1-936176-54-0

Printed in the United States

Notice: The authors and publisher have made every effort to ensure that the patient care recommended herein, including choice of drugs and drug dosages, is in accord with the accepted standard and practice at the time of publication. However, since research and regulation constantly change clinical standards, the reader is urged to check the product information sheet included in the package of each drug, which includes recommended doses, warnings, and contraindications. This is particularly important with new or infrequently used drugs. Any treatment regimen, particularly one involving medication, involves inherent risk that must be weighed on a case-by-case basis against the benefits anticipated. The reader is cautioned that the purpose of this book is to inform and enlighten; the information contained herein is not intended as, and should not be employed as, a substitute for individual diagnosis and treatment.

This fifth edition is dedicated to our teachers, mentors and our patients.

ABOUT THE AMERICAN ACADEMY OF ORAL MEDICINE (AAOM): The AAOM is a 501c6, nonprofit organization founded in 1945 as the American Academy of Dental Medicine and took its current name in 1966. The members of the American Academy of Oral Medicine include an internationally recognized group of health care professionals and experts concerned with the oral health care of patients who have complex medical conditions, oral mucosal disorders, and/or chronic orofacial pain. Oral Medicine is the field of dentistry concerned with the oral health care of medically complex patients and with the diagnosis and non-surgical management of medically-related disorders or conditions affecting the oral and maxillofacial region.

AMERICAN ACADEMY OF ORAL MEDICINE

MISSION:

1. To promote the study and dissemination of knowledge of the medical aspects of dentistry while serving the best interests of the public.

2. To promote the highest standards of care in the diagnosis and treatment of oral conditions that are not responsive to conventional dental or oral maxillofacial surgical procedures.

3. To provide an avenue of referral for dental practitioners who have patients with severe, life-threatening medical disorders or complex diagnostic problems involving the oral and maxillofacial region that require ongoing nonsurgical management.

4. To improve the quality of life of patients with medically related oral disease.

5. To foster increased understanding and cooperation between medical and dental professions.

6. To obtain American Dental Association recognition of oral medicine as a specialty.

The Academy achieves these goals by holding national meetings annually; by presenting lectures, workshops, and seminars; by sponsorship of the American Board of Oral Medicine; by the editorship of the Oral Medicine Section of *Oral Surgery, Oral Medicine, Oral Pathology, Oral Radiology*, and *Endodontology*; and by publishing monographs and position papers on timely subjects relating to oral medicine.

The presented information is based on current knowledge and accepted standards of practice. Following the guidelines set forth in this monograph may not ensure successful management of every patient. This monograph represents a consensus of the editors and authors and not necessarily the private views of any individual.

All brand name medications may have patents, service marks, trademarks, or registered trademarks and are the property of their respective companies.

This Clinician's Guide is another AAOM educational service.
Other Clinician's Guides available from the Academy include:

Oral Health in Geratric Patient 3/e
Treatment of Common Oral Conditions, 7/e
Tobacco Cessation, 2/e
Pharmacology in Dental Medicine, 2/e
Chronic Orofacial Pain, 4/e
Medically Complex Dental Patients 4/e

Preface

Human immunodeficiency virus (HIV) infection and acquired immune deficiency syndrome (AIDS) was first reported in 1981. In the most recent data available (2014) the Centers for Disease Control and Prevention (CDC) estimated over 1.1 million individuals in the United States (U.S.) were living with HIV; 15% were without knowledge of their diagnosis. The annual number of new HIV infections (incidence) in the U.S. has decreased over time and for the most recent data period 37, 600 Americans per year are diagnosed. Since the beginning of the epidemic the number of deaths attributed to AIDS in the U.S. is over 678, 509 people. According to the World Health Organization (WHO), between 2000 and 2016 new HIV infections fell by 39%, and HIV-related deaths fell by one third. WHO's most recent estimate is more than 36.7 million people are living with HIV. Yearly, there are an estimated 1.8 million newly acquired infections and 1 million deaths attributed to AIDS.

First introduced in 1996, highly active antiretroviral therapies (HAART), a milestone treatment paradigm utilizing three or more antiretroviral drugs used in combination, have improved the length and quality of life for HIV positive persons who have access to these medications. HIV has the ability to mutate and replicate even in the presence of antiretroviral drugs. This occurrence has lead to antiviral drug resistance and the spread of drug resistant strains of HIV. Consequently, new drugs and drug classes have been developed and, moreover, must continue to be developed to help combat viral mutation in HIV disease and provide effective therapies for treatment experienced individuals.

Other challenges in treatment of HIV include numerous health disparities in incidence and treatment outcomes among different population groups. Health disparity is defined as a difference that occurs by gender, race, ethnicity, education, income, disability, geographical location or sexual orientation. For example, of the total number of individuals diagnosed with HIV in 2015, Black/African Americans comprised 44.3% and Whites comprised 5.3%. For comparison, the 2010 U.S. Census data reports 12.6% of the U.S. population as Black/African American and 72.4% as White. Additionally, studies show that Black/African Americans tend to present with lower CD4 cell counts at diagnosis compared to Whites. Another disparity identified was the number of days between diagnosis of HIV and initiation of treatment. Black/African Americans were found on average to have 264 days between diagnosis and treatment compared with 102 days for Whites.

Gender disparity in HIV disease also exists. Data from large cohorts confirm that women with HIV are 1.5 times less likely to receive clinically indicated treatment. Moreover, female participation in clinical trials has not been to the same degree as male participation and there is emerging evidence that women are at increased risk for side effects from certain antiretroviral drugs.

Factors thought to be associated with these disparities are complex and may include unequal insurance coverage, access to medical services, and patterns of healthcare utilization. Viral mutation, HIV drug resistance and health disparities will provide challenges for prevention and treatment in the coming decade.

Treatment modalities for HIV disease are changing rapidly aided by advancing technology. New treatment modalities, medications, laboratory parameters as well as available resources are continually added and updated.

This rapid growth and change of information has promoted an expansion of the traditional role of dental health care workers. The dental healthcare worker in the era of AIDS:

1. Provides routine dental care for HIV-positive individuals. HIV-positive patients can be safely treated by general dental practitioners as there are no complications associated with dental care that are more common among HIV-positive patients compared to HIV-negative patients.

2. Understands the significance of oral lesions associated with HIV disease, and performs evaluations, diagnostic assessment, and institutes treatment. Some oral lesions found in HIV-positive persons are reliable markers for immune suppression, disease progression and AIDS diagnosis.

3. Collaborates with other health care workers and social support systems involved in the overall care of HIV-positive patients. Overall care for HIV-positive patients will improve when more health care workers can perform adequate oral examinations and distinguish between normal and abnormal oral tissues.

▶▶ **Preface** *continued*

4. Becomes involved in HIV-related education for other health care workers and the lay community. Educating non-HIV-positive patients on the facts associated with HIV transmission and treatment of the disease by dental healthcare workers should lessen fear concerning this disease. This lessened fear of the disease transmission should lead to decreased discrimination toward HIV-positive individuals.

5. Acts as a resource to HIV-positive colleagues. HIV-positive dental health care workers need support from their peers in order to better cope with their disease.

Viral hepatitis is the leading cause of hepatocellular carcinoma in the U.S. and the most common cause for liver transplantation. In the U.S., an estimated 850,000 Americans are living with chronic hepatitis B and 3.5 million are living with chronic Hepatitis C. Many of these individuals with chronic hepatitis are unaware that they are infected. Each year an estimated 21,000 become infected with hepatitis B, and 33,900 with hepatitis C.

There are few if any complications associated with providing dental care to HIV-positive patients and patients with hepatitis B or hepatitis C. Therefore general dentists are able to provide dental care for HIV-positive patients and patients with hepatitis with few exceptions.

This fifth edition of the Clinician's Guide to Treatment of Patients with HIV and Other Communicable Diseases is intended to assist oral healthcare workers in obtaining information essential to becoming an integral part of the healthcare treatment team for individuals with HIV, hepatitis and tuberculosis (TB). This monograph is provided as a reference for dental professionals treating persons living with these transmissible infectious diseases. The information is based on present knowledge and will change during the course of these epidemics. Management of any medically complex patients is a challenge and should always be governed with the patient's best interests in mind.

For the Editor and Contributors
Brian C. Muzyka, DMD, MS, MBA
January 2018

Standard Abbreviations

I	One	Prn	as needed (pro re nata)
ii	Two	Q	Every
iii	Three	q2h	every 2 hours
a	Before	q4h	every 4 hours
ac	before meals (ante cibum)	q6h	every 6 hours
ad lib	as desired (ad libitum)	q8h	every 8 hours
asap	as soon as possible	q12h	every 12 hours
AAOM	American Academy of Oral Medicine	Qam	every morning
bid	twice a day (bis in die)	Qd	every day (quaque die)
btl	Bottle	Qhs	every bedtime
c	With	Qid	four times a day (quarter in die)
cap	Capsule	Qod	every other day

Standard Abbreviations (continued)

CBC	complete blood count	Qpm	every evening
CDC	U. S. Center for Disease Control and Prevention	qsad	add a sufficient quantity to equal
crm	Cream	qwk	every week
disp	dispense on a prescription label	RAS	recurrent aphthous stomatitis
elix	Elixir	RAU	recurrent aphthous ulcer
FDA	U.S. Food and Drug Administration	RBC	red blood cell count
g	Gram	RHL	recurrent herpes labialis
gtt	Drop	RIH	recurrent intraoral herpes
h	Hour	Rx	Prescription
hs	at bedtime	s	Without
HSV	herpes simplex virus	Sig	patient dosing instructions on prescription label
IU	international units	Sol	Solution
IV	Intravenous	SPF	sun protection factor
L	Liter	stat	Immediately
liq	Liquid	Syr	Syrup
loz	Lozenge	Tab	Tablet
mg	Milligram	tbsp	Tablespoon
min	Minute	Tid	three times a day (ter in die)
mL	Milliliter	Top	Topical
NaF	sodium fluoride	Tsp	Teaspoon
Oint	Ointment	U	Unit
OTC	over-the-counter	ut dict	as directed (ut dictum)
Oz	Ounce	UV	Ultraviolet
P	After	Visc	Viscous
Pc	after meals	VZV	varicella-zoster virus
PABA	para-aminobenzoic acid	WBC	white blood cell count
PHN	postherpetic neuralgia	Wk	Week
PLT	platelet count	Yr	Year
Po	by mouth (per os)	Zn	Zinc

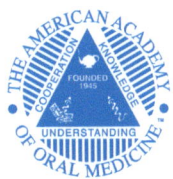

1 HIV Pathogenesis and Routes of Transmisison

Infection with HIV causes a progressive disease associated with immune dysregulation, dysfunction, and deficiency. Most patients with HIV disease (HIVD) left untreated will develop major opportunistic infections. These opportunistic infections can be associated with high morbidity and mortality as the immune response becomes increasingly impaired. Individuals with HIV may also develop various neoplasms such as Kaposi's sarcoma or non Hodgkin's lymphoma.

AIDS is the most advanced stage of HIV and is diagnosed when at least one of twenty-seven specific clinical disease entities, known as AIDS-defining illnesses (CDC 2008), is diagnosed. Additionally AIDS is also defined when a specific subset of T-lymphocytes expressing a CD4 membrane receptor (known as T4-helper lymphocytes or CD4+ cells) decline below a level of 200 cells/mm3 of (see Appendix A).

The pathogenesis of HIVD is based on interactions between the causative agent (HIV) and the host immune system. Cells expressing CD4 membrane receptors are the primary targets for HIV. Besides T4-helper lymphocytes, monocytes and macrophages also express these CD4 receptors, although to a lesser extent. The monocytes may serve as carriers for HIV, transporting the virus from lymphoid tissues to different parts of the body.

The most dramatic effect of HIV disease is observed when high levels of HIV replication occur in CD4+ lymphocytes, resulting in continual destruction of these lymphocytes. CD4+ lymphocytes lose their normal immune protective functions and ultimately are reduced in numbers. Consequently, the decline of CD4+ cell number and function is closely associated with the development of opportunistic oral and systemic infections. CD4+ cell counts in combination with HIV viral load levels (a measure of HIV RNA found in blood) are the most reliable predictors of disease progression and prognosis.

The main routes of HIV transmission in the U.S. are through unprotected anal and vaginal sex, and sharing of needles among injection drug users. Transmission through contaminated blood, blood products, and organ transplantation is extremely rare in the U.S. due to the rigorous screening of donors and testing of the U.S. blood supply and donated organs/tissue. Similarly, while transmission of HIV may also occur from an infected mother to her child during pregnancy or at birth, this mode of transmission is much less common since the U.S. Public Health Service guidelines for use of antiretroviral therapy for pregnant women and newborn infants (1994), and universal counseling and voluntary HIV testing of pregnant women (1995).

The natural history of HIV disease can be altered by effective medical management using highly active antiretroviral therapy (HAART). HAART employs combinations of antiretroviral drugs that target various steps of viral cell replication, (e.g., reverse transcription and assembly/release), thereby interrupting the cycle of HIV production within the CD4+ lymphocyte.

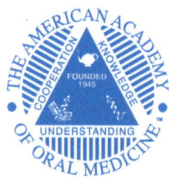

2 HIV Epidemiology And Trends

In 2008, the U.S. CDC revised the existing HIV case definition from 1993 to the following combined surveillance and case definitions for adults, adolescents and children over age 18 months:

HIV Infection, Stage Unknown:
No information available on CD4+ T-lymphocyte count or percentage and no information available on AIDS-defining conditions.

HIV Infection, Stage 1:
No AIDS-defining condition and either CD4+ T-lymphocyte count of >500 cells/µL or CD4+ T-lymphocyte percentage of total lymphocytes of >29.

HIV Infection, Stage 2:
No AIDS-defining condition and either CD4+ T-lymphocyte count of 200 – 499 cells/µL or CD4+ T-lymphocyte percentage of total lymphocytes of 14 – 28.

HIV Infection, Stage 3 (AIDS):
CD4+ T-lymphocyte count of <200 cells/µL or CD4+ T-lymphocyte percentage of total lymphocytes of <14 or documentation of an AIDS-defining condition. Documentation of an AIDS-defining condition supersedes a CD4+ T-lymphocyte count of >200 cells/µL and a CD4+ T-lymphocyte percentage of total lymphocytes of >14.

Laboratory confirmed presence of HIV is required for defining HIV. For surveillance purposes, HIV disease progression is classified from less to more severe; once cases are classified into a surveillance severity stage, they cannot be reclassified into a less severe stage although a subsequent laboratory or clinical marker may change.

The cumulative number of persons in the United States with diagnosed HIV infection ever classified as stage 3 (AIDS) at year-end 2015 was 1,216,917. The cumulative estimated number of deaths of persons with diagnosed HIV infection ever classified as stage 3 (AIDS) in the United States, through 2014, was 678,509.

In 2014, there were 12,333 AIDS deaths (due to any cause) and 6,721 deaths were attributed directly to HIV.

Since April 2008 all U.S. states and the six dependent U.S. territoties (American Samoa, Guam, Northern Mariana Islands, Puerto Rico, U.S. Virgin Islands) report HIV findings to the CDC. At the end of 2014, an estimated 1.1 million persons aged 13 and older in the U.S. were living with HIV infection, including an estimated 166,000 (15% of the total) persons whose infections had not been diagnosed. In the U.S more males are diagnosed with HIV/AIDS. Approximately 80% of the cumulative AIDS diagnosis in the U.S were males. Approximately 20% of the cumulative AIDS diagnosed were women.

Further classification of individuals diagnosed with AIDS by transmission category can be found in Table 2.1 on the following page.

EPIDEMIOLOGY OF HIV-RELATED ORAL DISEASE OVER THE PAST THREE DECADES
Since the onset of the AIDS epidemic in the 1980s, the oral cavity has had an important role in the natural history of HIV infection and AIDS. Specific oral lesions have served as an early hallmark for HIV/AIDS and for monitoring disease progression.

Hairy leukoplakia, a white corrugated non removable Epstein-Barr virus related plaque usually on the lateral border of the tongue, was first noted in San Francisco in 1984. A number of other mucosal diseases were found to affect the oral cavity of severely immunosuppressed people, most of which were opportunistic infections associated with various fungal and viral pathogens (e.g., candidiasis, warts,

TABLE 2-1: CUMULATIVE ESTIMATE OF AIDS BY TRANSMISSION CATEGORY IN THE UNITED STATES			
Transmission Category	Cumulative Estimated # of AIDS Diagnoses, Through 2014*		
	Adult and Adolescent Males	**Adult and Adolescent Females**	**Total**
Male-to-male sexual contact	589,764	–	589,764
Injection drug use	186,426	90,7229	277,148
Male-to-male sexual contact and injection drug use	86,3315	–	86,331
Heterosexual contact**	85,011	151,561	236,572
Other***	11,649	5,987	17,636
Total			1,207,451

* From the beginning of the epidemic through 2014.
** Heterosexual contact with a person known to have, or to be at high risk for, HIV infection.
*** Includes hemophilia, blood transfusion, perinatal exposure, and risk not reported or not identified.

Centers for Disease Control and Prevention. HIV Surveillance Report, 2015; vol. 27.
http://www.cdc.gov/hiv/library/reports/hiv-surveillance.html. Published November 2016.

and recurrent herpes simplex infections). While some bacterial infections (e.g., necrotizing ulcerative gingivitis, periodontitis, and necrotizing stomatitis) and neoplasms (e.g., Kaposi sarcoma and non-Hodgkin's lymphoma) were also observed, they were less common. Epidemiologic studies conducted in the late 1980s and early 1990s revealed that oral candidiasis and hairy leukoplakia were the most common lesions found in the oral cavity, and their occurrence has been shown to be strongly associated with a low CD4+ cell count and a higher plasma viral load. In populations with more advanced HIV disease (i.e., CD4+ cell count < 200 cells/mm3 , AIDS), the prevalence of oral candidiasis ranged from 30 to 70% and that of hairy leukoplakia from 19 to 38%. Other oral lesions such as warts, non-specific ulcers, and Kaposi sarcoma rarely exceeded 5%.

With the advent of combination highly active antiretroviral therapy (HAART), the prevalence of HIV-related oral lesions has decreased significantly. In one prospective study in Spain, the prevalence of oral candidiasis decreased from 31% prior to initiation of HAART to 1% 48 weeks after initiation of HAART. In another study

in the U.S., the prevalence of hairy leukoplakia when comparing a population before and after the advent of HAART was found to be 26 and 11%, respectively. However, other conditions such as oral warts and salivary gland disease may be more common in a HAART population. In a retrospective study of 1,280 HIV-positive patients visiting an oral medicine clinic in San Francisco from 1990 to 1999, investigators found a statistically significantly higher proportion of individuals with oral warts among those on HAART (23%) than among those who were not on therapy (5%). The reason for this possible increase in the prevalence of warts among people receiving HAART is not clear. A study published in 2012 noted oral HPV infection in HIV-negative individuals were associated with *recent* number of oral sex partners but in HIV-positive individuals oral HPV infections were associated with *lifetime* number of oral sex partners and current CD4. These differences are consistent with the hypothesis that prevalent oral HPV infections may represent primarily recently acquired infection among HIV-negative adults but in HIV-positive adults may be more likely to represent persistent or previously acquired reactivated oral HPV infections.

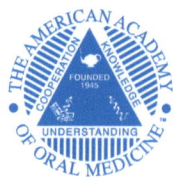

3 HIV Clinical Disease Course

INCUBATION PERIOD AND SURVIVAL

The median incubation period of HIV, from initial infection to the first clinical signs and symptoms of AIDS, is approximately 10 years when patients do not receive effective medical management (i.e. combination HAART). The estimate varies with the age at which infection occurs and is significantly shorter in infants and in older adults. Determining whether the incubation period varies by mode of HIV transmission has been more difficult to determine. The majority of evidence now indicates that, after adjustment for age, the incubation period is similar in injecting drug users, those infected sexually, and hemophiliacs. Incubation time in transfusion recipients is shorter, most likely because of the large HIV inoculum in infected blood. The incubation period does not appear to vary significantly in men and women or in different racial groups. Reasons for the shortened AIDS incubation period may include failure to diagnose HIV infection or lack of access or adherence to medications and supportive timely medical care among those with known HIV disease.

Response to combination HAART has dramatically prolonged the incubation period of HIV-positive individuals to AIDS regardless of their HIV transmission risk. The prolonged AIDS incubation period for HIV results in delaying diagnoses of AIDS. New therapies have converted HIV infection into a chronic manageable disease.

Presently a cure for HIV is not available and an effective vaccine is not likely to be developed in the near future. The evolution of antiretroviral drug resistant strains of HIV, and individuals carrying and transmitting these resistant strains, have rendered certain medications in our current treatment repertoire ineffective for controlling HIV replication in the newly infected. New pharmacologic approaches to attack HIV during other phases of its lifecycle, such as entry inhibitors or fusion inhibitors, are available and others are under investigation.

Furthermore, with initiation of combination HAART, many individuals with a history of AIDS-associated illnesses may have at least a partially restored immune system which can help protect against subsequent episodes of opportunistic infections. Additionally, there are clearly defined subpopulations of HIV-positive individuals who survive (long-term survivors) and do not show signs of HIV disease progression for long periods of time (long-term non-progressors) even in the absence of HAART.

MEDICAL HISTORY

Health questionnaires used in the dental office should include pertinent questions in order to assess a patient's medical status prior to dental therapy. HIV disease is now a chronic illness and as with all chronic diseases, frequent updates of the patient's medical history are essential. The patient's past and present medical status should be reviewed when determining appropriate dental therapy. Medical status information, along with input from the patient will influence the formulation of a treatment plan consistent with the expectations and needs of the patient.

It is important to recognize that modifications to the patient's dental therapy are based on the patient's overall medical status. A patient's HIV status and disease progression may indicate possible medical conditions.

Table 3-1 includes significant information relevant to the initial and ongoing assessment of patients at risk for and those living with HIV.

TABLE 3-1: CATEGORIES TO CONSIDER WHEN ASSESSING HIV-POSITIVE PATIENTS FOR DENTAL TREATMENT			
Category	**Considerations**		
First, subsequent and current HIV RNA (viral load)	Will help to determine viremia, adherence to HAART, development of drug resistance		
First, subsequent and current CD4+ cell count	Will help to determine immune status, disease progression, AIDS diagnosis if <200, and prognosis		
Past and present HIV-related opportunistic infections	Indicates past and present immune status, disease state, progression, and medications		
Past history of sexually transmitted diseases (STDs).	Frequent episodes of STDs are associated with increased disease progression	Past infections with syphilis may result in neurosyphilis and cardiomyopathies	
Past and present history of other diseases	Chronic infection with HBV, HCV and HDV may result in liver disease and may accelerate HIV progression	Exposure to TB and length of time on anti-tuberculocidal medication may indicate infectious TB status	Noncompliance with anti-TB medications may result in multidrug resistant TB (MDR-TB)
Medications	Indicate past and present HIV-related conditions, immune status, and disease progression	Indicate possible hematologic abnormalities.	Medications may have oral side effects that require management or increase the risk of drug interactions with drugs prescribed by the dentist
Allergies	Increased incidence of adverse effects to medications during disease progression		
Social History	Alcohol use may enhance HIV replication. Alcohol may cause drug interactions	Injection drug users need to be counseled. Substance abuse associated with high risk behaviors	Tobacco use may increase incidence of oral candidiasis
Laboratory values	Higher incidence of anemia, granulocytopenia and thrombocytopenia	Evaluation of level of viremia and immune status	Indicate need for consultations and possible premedication or blood transfusion support
Review of systems			
Head and neck	Lymphadenopathy	Sinusitis	
Dermatology	Facial lesions may be contagious		
Gastrointestinal	Wasting syndrome	Hepatitis	Splenectomy
Pulmonary	Tuberculosis		
Neurologic Manifestations	Cognitive and motor impairments	Neuropathies	Dementia

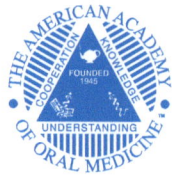

4 **HIV Medications and Implications for Dentistry**

Traditional treatment for HIV and AIDS consists of differing classes of medications given to control viral replication. Currently the U.S. Food and Drug Administration (FDA) recognizes 7 classes of drugs.

Specific information regarding side effects, dosages and indications should be reviewed from a comprehensive drug index. The seven classes of drugs used in management of HIV viral replication are: nucleoside reverse transcriptase inhibitors (NRTI), non-nucleoside reverse transcriptase inhibitors (NNRTI), protease inhibitors (PI), fusion inhibitors (FI), entry inhibitors (EI), Integrase Strand Transfer Inhibitors (INSTI), pharmokinetic enhancers, and multiclass combination products.

TABLE 4-1: HIV MEDICATIONS AND IMPLICATIONS FOR DENTISTRY		
Brand name	**Generic Name**	**Oral Side effects**
Multi-class Combination products		
Atripla	Efavirenz, emtricitabine and tenofovir disoproxil fumarate	Throat irritation, erythema multiforme (rare)
Nucleoside Reverse Transcriptase Inhibitors (NRTIs)		
Combivir	Lamivudine and zidovudine	See Lamivudine and Zidovudine
Emtriva	Emtricitabine, (FTC)	Nasopharyngitis
Epivir	Lamivudine, (3TC)	Stomatitis\
Epzicom	Abacavir and lamivudine	Pharyngitis, stomatitis
Retrovir	Zidovudine, azidothymidine	Bleeding gingiva, dysphagia, edema of the tongue, mouth ulcer, oral mucosa pigmentation, taste perversion have been reported in patients receiving zidovudine
Trizivir	Abacavir, zidovudine, and lamivudine	See Lamivudine and Zidovudine
Truvada	Tenofovir disoproxil fumarate and emtricitabine,	See emtricitabine
Videx EC	Enteric coated dideoxyinosine, (ddl EC)	Dry mouth sialadenitis
Viread	Tenofovir disoproxil fumarate, (TDF)	
Zerit	Stavudine, (d4T)	
Ziagen	Abacavir sulfate, (ABC)	Mouth ulcerations, pharyngitis

TABLE 4-1: HIV MEDICATIONS AND IMPLCATIONS FOR DENTISTRY (continued)		
Brand name	*Generic Name*	*Oral Side effects*
Nonnucleoside Reverse Transcriptase Inhibitors (NNRTIs)		
Edurant	Rilpivirine	
Intelence	Etravirine	Erythema multforme
Rescriptor	Delavirdine, (DLV)	Dry mouth, dysphagia, bleeding gingiva, stomatitis, taste perversion, tongue edema, toothache
Sustiva	Efavirenz, (EFV)	Stomatitis
Viramune	Nevirapine, (NVP)	Stomatitis
Protease Inhibitors (PI)		
Agenerase	Amprenavir, (APV)	Taste perversion
Aptivus	Tipranavir, (TPV)	
Crixivan	Indinavir, (IDV)	
Invirase	Saquinavir mesylate, (SQV)	
Kaletra	Lopinavir and ritonavir, (LPV/RTV)	Dry mouth
Lexiva	Fosamprenavir calcium, (FOS-APV)	
Norvir	Ritonavir, (RTV)	Taste perversion
Prezista	Darunavir	Pharyngitis, dry mouth
Reyataz	Atazanavir sulfate, (ATV)	Oral ulcers
Viracept	Nelfinavir mesylate, (NFV)	Pharyngitis, oral ulcers
Fusion Inhibitors (FI)		
Fuzeon	Enfuvirtide, (T-20)	Taste perversions, dry mouth
Entry Inhibitors CCR5 co-receptor Antagonist (EI)		
Selzentry	Maraviroc	
HIV Integrase Strand Transfer Inhibitors (INSTI)		
Isentress	Raltegravir	
Tivicay	Dolutegravir	
Vitekta	Elvitegravir	
Pharmakinetic Enhancers		
Tybost	Cobicistat	

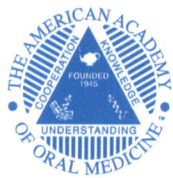

5 HIV Pertinent Laboratory Tests

HIV TESTING

The most commonly used HIV tests detect HIV antibodies (see below). On average most people will develop detectable HIV antibodies within 25 days (range 2 to 8 weeks) of their infection. Ninety-seven percent of persons will develop detectable antibodies in the first 3 months and rarely may take up to 6 months. The period of time from infection until detection is known as the "window period" and varies between individuals. During the window period HIV viral load may be very high and therefore more likely transmitted via unprotected sex and sharing of needles.

There are several serologic tests for evaluating HIV status. In order for an individual to be considered HIV positive, two consecutive Enzyme-linked immunosorbent assay (ELISA) tests followed by one Western Blot test must be positive for antibodies to HIV.

Antibody Tests:

Enzyme-linked immunosorbent assay (ELISA/EIA) – Detects a general antibody response to HIV. Most rapid HIV antibody tests, that give results in 10-20 minutes from blood or oral fluids, are considered screening tests and are based on a single ELISA/EIA.

Western blot (WB) – Detects antibody response to specific HIV proteins.

Antigen Tests:

p24 antigen – This test is no longer routinely used in the U.S. or Europe. The test detects HIV replication even prior to the formation of antibodies and can be used to detect infection during the "window period." Nucleic Acid testing (NAT) is more commonly used for detecting virus during the window period.

Nucleic Acid Tests:

Nucleic acid testing allows very small amounts of genetic material such as DNA or RNA to be copied and tested.

NAT has been used since 2001 in the U.S. to screen blood donations for HIV and HCV. Advantages of using NAT are that the window period is reduced to 12–16 days. Examples of NAT include reverse transcription polymerase chain reaction (RT-PCR) and branch DNA (bDNA) testing.

Measurement of HIV RNA as a disease monitoring tool will be addressed in the next section.

HIV TESTING PROCEDURE

In 2006, the CDC began advocating an HIV prevention plan for the U.S. that involves "opt out" testing. The CDC plan recommended all 13 to 64 year old patients in U.S. healthcare settings undergo non-targeted screening for HIV. Thus patients would be tested without regard to real or perceived risk for HIV and additionally without regard to signs or symptoms of HIV infection. This plan proposes state law be changed such that HIV testing is explicitly included in general consent to treat patients and thus specific refusal of consent for HIV testing is needed. Some state laws have changed to endorse this plan. However, some U.S. states and territories still require pre- and post-test counseling before performing "opt in" HIV testing. Failure to counsel, when required by state law, may result in legal actions. Knowledge of state law pertinent to HIV testing and confidentiality is important for the provider. Further information regarding state HIV testing laws can be found o the CDC website (https://www.cdc.gov/hiv/policies/law/states/index.html). Although most HIV testing is performed on blood specimens, a variety of testing sites and screening and testing modalities are available including rapid tests, oral mucosal transudate-based tests, home test systems, and traditional point of care testing in health departments, physician offices, drug treatment centers, prisons, STD clinics, prenatal clinics, and blood donation centers.

INDICATIONS FOR HIV TESTING OF DENTAL PATIENTS

If agreeable, dental patients should be referred to a physician for evaluation and confidential HIV testing when

TABLE 5-1: CLINICAL IMPACT OF CD4 COUNT REDUCTION IN ADULTS AND ADOLESCENTS		
CD4 cells/mm³	**CD4 %**	**Clinical Impact**
>600	32-50	Normal value.
<500	<29	Initial immune suppression.
<400		Manifestations of opportunistic infections, including oral lesions.
200-400	14-28	Increased number and severity of opportunistic infections.
<200	<14	Severe immune suppression. Appearance of major opportunistic infections. Initiation of prophylactic medications for PCP. AIDS diagnosis.
<100		Appearance of fatal opportunistic infections, neoplasms and specific oral lesions. Initiation of prophylactic medication for toxoplasmosis, MAC and cryptococcosis.

clinical manifestations raise suspicion of HIV disease. Alternatively, the dentist can use a point of care oral fluids test, such as Oraquick ADVANCE® HIV-1/2 rapid antibody test (Orasure Technologies, Inc., Bethlehem, PA) to screen for HIV antibodies. If this is positive, then the dentist should facilitate ready access to confirmatory testing, counseling and medical care follow-up. Post exposure needlestick protocols may include requests for patients to be tested for HIV. Involuntary testing of patient's blood can be court ordered when an occupational exposure has occurred, according to specific state laws.

PERTINENT LABORATORY TESTS AND VALUES

CD4 cell count: (Normal 544-1663; median 935). This test measures the number (cells/mm³) of peripheral T4 (helper)-lymphocytes.

CD4 %: (Normal 32-60%; median 46%). This test measures the percent of CD4+ cells of total lymphocytes. The CD4 % is less subject to variation on repeated measurements.

> CD4 counts usually will determine disease stage and may influence treatment planning. There is no need for prophylactic medication for dental therapy based solely on CD4 cell status.

CD8 cell count: (Normal 272-932; median 519). This test measures the number (cells/mm³) of peripheral T8 (suppressor)-lymphocytes. These cells have been implicated in suppression of HIV. High numbers of CD8 cells may be beneficial to the patient.

Viral load: Measurement of viral replication of HIV (viremia) in blood plasma. Range of detection is from < 50 copies/ml to 10,000,000 copies/ml of HIV-1. The highest

peripheral blood viral load is generally found during the first 3 months after initial infection and during the late stages of the disease. In the absence of ART, there is usually stable plasma and cellular viremia during the asymptomatic stage of disease. Less than 10,000 copies/ml of HIV mRNA in plasma indicates slow HIV progression. Viral load measurement is intended for use in conjunction with clinical presentation and other laboratory markers of disease progress for the clinical management of HIV positive patients. The goal of HAART is obtaining and maintaining an undetectable viral load.

Secondary to treatment with HAART, decreases in *community viral load*, a mathematical measure of the amount of virus in a particular population, were associated with a decrease in the number of new HIV diagnoses in San Francisco, California, between 2004 and 2008. Increasing HAART to a near as 100% as possible benefits the entire community through a reduction of HIV transmission.

> Viral load will determine level of viremia, efficacy of antiretroviral therapy, disease progression, and prognosis, and influences appropriate treatment planning. There is no need for prophylactic medication prior to dental therapy based solely on viral load.

Platelet count: (Normal 150,000 – 400,000 platelets/mm³). Thrombocytopenia (<150,000 platelets/mm³) may be present in 9% to 13% of asymptomatic HIV patients and 21% to 43% of adults with AIDS. Severe thrombocytopenia is rare, with <50,000 platelets/mm³ occurring in <1% of HIV positive patients.

Dental treatments, including extractions, can be safely performed in patients with platelet counts >50,000 platelets/mm³.

White blood cell count (WBC) and differential: (Normal WBC: 4,500 – 10,000 cells/mm³; neutrophils: 43-77% or 2,500 – 7,000 cells/mm³; lymphocytes: 21-35% or 1,000 – 4,800 cells/mm³; monocytes: 0-9% or 0 – 800 cells/mm³.) Leukopenia (white blood cell count below 4,500 cells/mm³) is present in 8% to 22% of asymptomatic HIV patients and 58% to 65% of patients with AIDS. This is due mainly to a decreased lymphocyte cell count. Neutrophil cell count may be low during the more advanced stages of the disease.

Prophylactic bactericidal antibiotics should be considered when the neutrophil count is below 500 cells/mm³ (normal 2,500-7,000 cells/mm³). When neutrophil counts are 500 cells/mm³ or less, patients are often already medicated with antibiotics due to frequent bacterial infections and as prophylaxis against opportunistic infections.

Hemoglobin: Many HIV patients are anemic, both secondary to medications and as a direct result of the HIV infection. Many patients present with hemoglobin (HgB) levels of 7.0 g/dl to 10.0 g/dl (normal: males 14 g/dl to 18 g/dl; females 12 g/dl to 16 g/dl). It is important to establish a baseline value for each individual and correlate subsequent hemoglobin levels with the baseline value.

PT/INR and PTT: Normal values of prothrombin time (PT) (less than 2 seconds deviation from control, usually 9-11 seconds)/International Normalized Ratio (INR) (1.0), and partial thromboplastin time (PTT) (28-38 seconds) usually indicate absence of liver damage and inherited coagulation disorders, such as hemophilia.

There are no contraindications for general dental procedures, including single extractions, for patients with normal bleeding time and coagulation values up to double the normal values and hemoglobin levels above 7.0 g/dl. Avoid respiratory depressant drugs with hemoglobin levels below 10 g/dl.

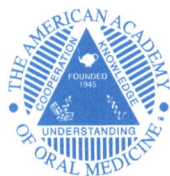

6 HIV Common Oral Manifestations and Management

DIAGNOSIS AND MANAGEMENT

Standardized case-definitions for common HIV-related oral lesions have been published as part of the Oral HIV/AIDS Research Alliance. The following case-definitions are adapted from the most recent publication (July 2009).

FUNGAL INFECTIONS

Pseudomembranous candidiasis

Case definition: White or yellow/creamy spots or plaques that may be located in any part of the oral cavity and can usually be wiped off to reveal an erythematous surface (Figures 6-1a and 6-1b). Patient may report no or mild to moderate burning pain. Lesions/symptoms are usually intermittent, but may be long-standing.

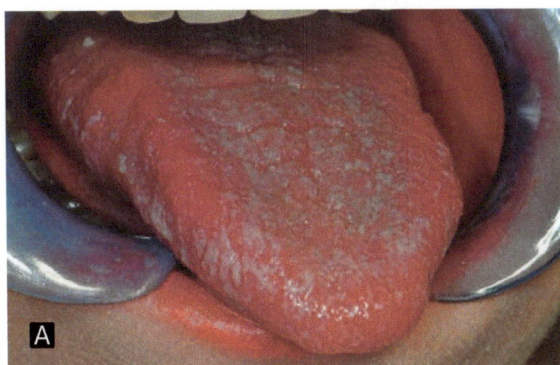

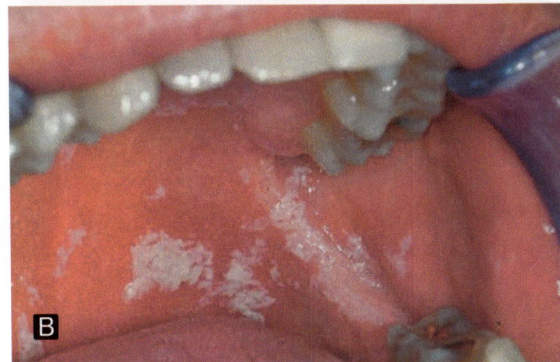

FIGURES 6-1a and 6-1b: *Pseudomembranous candidiasis, tongue (a) and left soft palate and retromolar area (b).*

Management: Both topical and systemic agents are available and effective for the treatment of oral candidiasis, and the selection of either type of agent (topical versus systemic is based on: 1) severity and extent of disease; and 2) other medications currently taken by patient (e.g., azoles potentiate cyclosporine and a number of antidiabetic medications, and is contra-indicated among patients taking warfarin, statins increase risk for myopathy). Treatment duration is usually 14 days.

Topical antifungals:

> **Rx**: Clotrimazole troches (10 mg)
> Disp: 70
> Sig: Dissolve 1 troche in mouth 5 times per day

> **Rx**: Nystatin (vaginal troches) 100,000u
> Disp: 56
> Sig: Dissolve 1 troche in mouth 4 times per day

> **Rx**: Miconazole mucobuccal tablet (50 mg) (Oravig®)
> Disp: 14
> Sig: Apply one tablet once daily to upper gum and allow to slowly dissolve during the day

Systemic antifungals:

> **Rx**: Fluconazole tabs 100m
> Disp: 15
> Sig: Take 2 tabs stat, then 1 tab daily

> **Rx**: Itraconazole caps 100mgs
> Disp: 28
> Sig: Take 2 caps after meals

Erythematous candidiasis

Case definition: Patchy erythema or red areas usually located on the palate and dorsum of the tongue, but occasionally on the buccal mucosa. At times, white spots or plaques of pseudomembranous candidiasis may also be present (Figures 2a and 2b). Patient may report no or mild to moderate burning pain. Lesions/symptoms are usually intermittent, but may be long-standing.

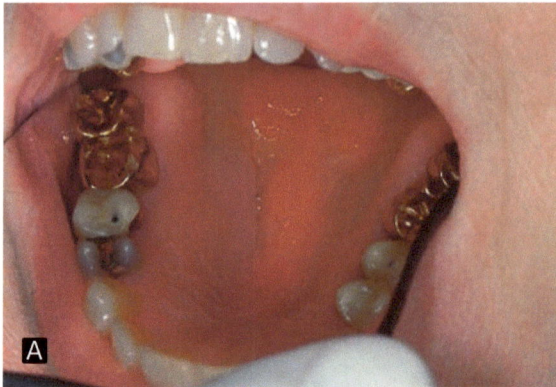

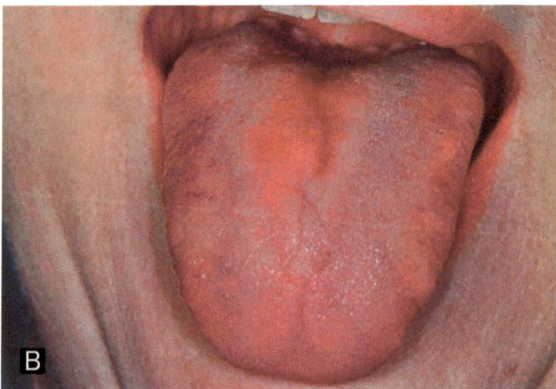

FIGURES 6-2a and 6-2b: *Erythematous candidiasis, palate (a) and dorsum of tongue (b).*

Management: Erythematous candidasis is managed the same as for pseudomembranous candidiasis.

Angular cheilitis

Case definition: Red or white fissures or linear ulcers located at the lip commissures or corners of the mouth (Figure 6-3). Patient may report no or mild pain when opening his/her mouth. Lesions/symptoms are usually intermittent, but may be long-standing.

Management: Angular cheilitis is managed the same as for pseudomembra-nous candidiasis, even if there is no evidence of intra-oral candidiasis, with topical appli-cations of an antifungal cream or ointment. Note that if angular cheilitis is severe and does not clear with antifun-gal treatment, one should consider secondary bacterial

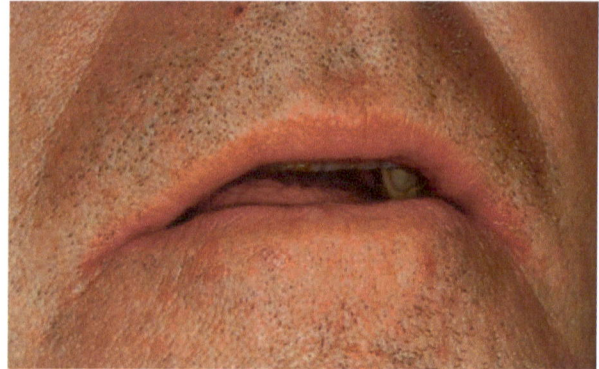

FIGURE 6-3: *Angular cheilitis*

colonization, and application of mupirocin ointment 2% three times daily (disp: 15 gm) may be useful in addition to the antifungal ointment or cream.

Topical antifungal cream/ointments:

> **Rx:** Clotrimazole ointment 1%, miconazole ointment 2%, ketoconazole 2% cream, nystatin ointment; nystatin 100,000 u/gm and triamcinolone 0.1% ointment or cream
> Disp: Most agents available in 15 gm tube
> Sig: Apply to affected tissue 4 times per day

VIRAL INFECTIONS

Hairy leukoplakia

Case definition: Whitish/grey lesions on the lateral margins of the tongue. They are not removable and may exhibit vertical corrugations. Lesions range in size as they may be less than one centimeter, or may extend onto the ventral and dorsal surfaces of the tongue where they are usually flat. They may be bilateral or unilateral (Figure 6-4). Lesions are asymptomatic, and usually long-standing.

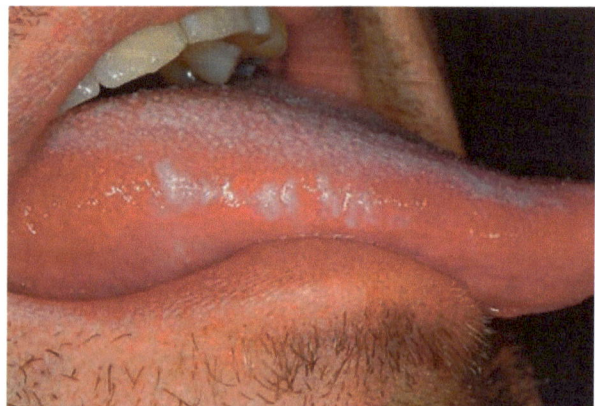

FIGURE 6-4: *Hairy leukoplakia right lateral tongue*

Management: Hairy leukoplakia is usually not treated because it is asymptomatic and there is no known risk of malignant transformation.

Exceptionally, lesions may be particularly thick and be an esthetic concern for the patient. The first step would be to treat the patient with an antifungal as secondary fungal colonization may be a possibility. If lesions remain thick and esthetically displeasing, topical applications of podophyllin may be useful. High dose acyclovir (800 mg four times daily for 10 days) may also be effective, but lesions usually recur after a few months.

Note: If lesion is unilateral, biopsy may be indicated to distinguish it from idiopathic leukoplakia.

Recurrent herpes simplex virus (HSV) infection
Case definition: Recurrent Herpes labialis presents as single or multiple vesicles or ulcers with crusting on vermillion portion of lips and adjacent facial skin (Figure 6-5a). Recurrent Intra-oral herpes simplex presents as solitary, or cluster of multiple or confluent ulcers that may be noted together with vesicles on keratinized mucosa, including hard palate, attached gingiva, and dorsum of tongue. Round to slightly irregular (map-like) margins with

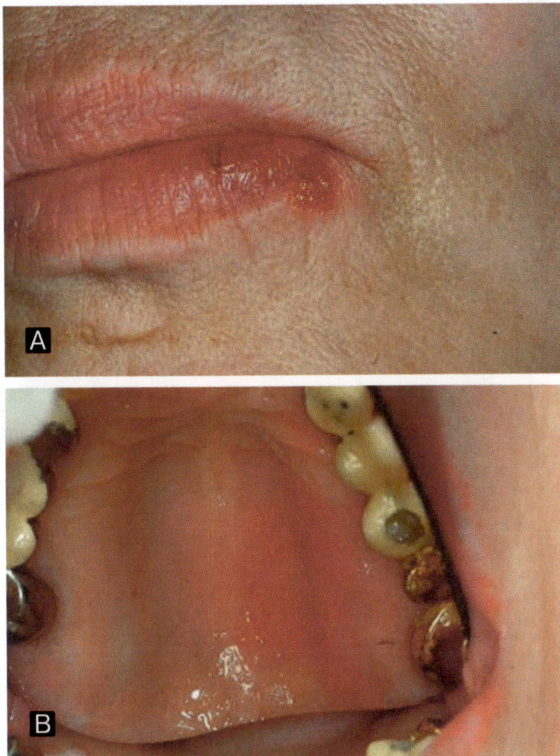

FIGURES 6-5a and 6-5b: *Herpes labialis, lower left vermilion border (a) and recurrent intraoral herpes infection, hard palate (b).*

minimal to no erythematous halos are present. The base of the ulcers is usually pink (Figure 6-5b). Patient usually reports mild to moderate pain, and prior history of (or recurrent) lesion(s). Lesion(s) are usually present for at most 10-14 days.

Management: While palliative care only is usually recommended in the immune competent host, treatment with a herpes-specific antiviral drug is recommended in the immunosuppressed patient, and should be initiated as early as possible after onset to significantly reduce the duration of the episode.

Rx: Acyclovir tabs 800 mg
Disp: 50
Sig: Take 1 tab 4 times per day for 10 days

Rx: Valacyclovir caplets 1000 mg
Disp: 20
Sig: Take 1 caplet 2 times daily for 10 days

Oral warts
Case definition: Mucosal color or white, solitary or multiple (often clustered) raised lesions that range in texture as they may be smooth, spiky, or cauliflower-like, and located in any part of the oral cavity (Figure 6-6). Usually asymptomatic, although warts on the buccal or labial mucosa or tongue may get traumatized by biting, and may be painful. Lesion(s) are usually long-standing.

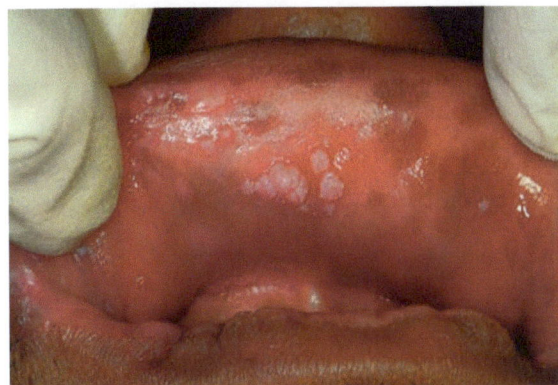

FIGURE 6-6: *Warts, upper labial mucosa*

Management: A biopsy is recommended as warts may be dysplastic. (The biopsy will usually reveal the presence of viral inclusions as warts are caused by the Human Papilloma Virus or HPV.) There is no effective predictable treatment for oral warts as they often recur after excision.

Selective excision should be performed on warts affecting areas that are either esthetically displeasing (e.g., lips, commissures), or interfere with function (e.g., buccal and labial mucosa). The CO2 laser (with high speed evacuation) is useful when warts have a broad base or are clustered, but scalpel excision is appropriate for isolated warts. Application of condylox gel 0.5% may be somewhat helpful. The usual schedule is twice a day for 3 days, followed by 4 days without treatment. This cycle may be repeated for up to 4 weeks.

IDIOPATHIC CONDITIONS

Recurrent Aphthous stomatitis

Case definition: Single or multiple, white/yellow well circumscribed ulcer(s) on non-keratinized tissue. A red hallo is usually present around each ulcer. Minor aphthous ulcers may be 0.2 to 0.5 cm in diameter (Figure 6-7a) and always appear on non-keratinized mucosa, while major aphthous ulcers are > 0.5 cm (may be as large as 2 cm in diameter), and may affect both keratinized and non-keratinized mucosa (Figure 6-7b). Patient may report moderate pain, especially upon eating, with minor aphthous ulcers, while severe pain is characteristic of major aphthous ulcers. Minor aphthous ulcers usually last 7-10 days, while major aphthous ulcers may last for weeks. In recurrent aphthous patient's report a long-term history of recurrent ulcers.

Management: The use of a topical steroid compound or a rinse is useful in accelerating the healing of aphthous ulcers. The patient should also be instructed to use a mild toothpaste without sodium-lauryl-sulfate, whitening agents, or tartar-control agents. In the case of major aphthous ulcers, because secondary bacterial colonization of the ulcer is often present, it is important to treat these ulcers with a topical antibacterial agent in addition to the topical steroid compound. If major aphthous ulcers do not respond to topical treatment, a short course of high-dose prednisone (60 mg/daily) for 5 days may be effective, but the patient's primary care provider should be consulted prior to administering a corticosteroid to an immunosuppressed patient. Any ulcer not responding to therapy within 2-3 weeks should be biopsied to rule out malignancy.

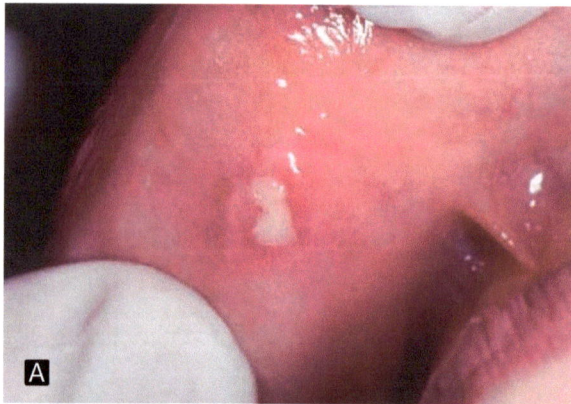

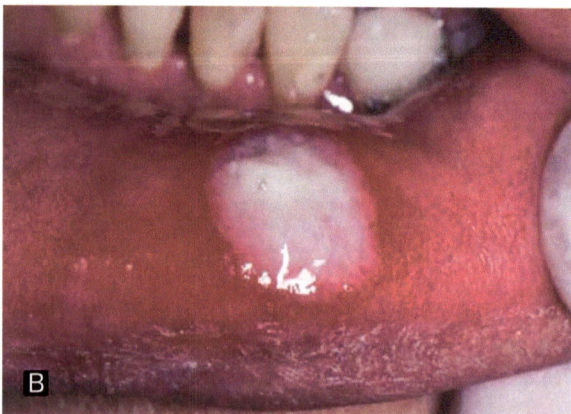

FIGURES 6-7a and 6-7b: *Minor aphthous ulcer, right buccal mucosa (a) and major aphthous ulcer, lower labial mucosa (b)*

Topical treatment of minor recurrent aphthous ulcers:

Rx: Fluocinonide (or clobetasol) ointment 0.05% to be mixed 50/50 with 20% benzocaine paste
Disp: 30 gm
Sig: Apply to ulcers 3 times per day

Rx: Dexamethasone solution 0.5mg/5mL
Disp: 250 mL
Sig: Rinse for 1 minute then expectorate 3 times per day

Topical treatment of major recurrent aphthous ulcers:

Rx: Tetracycline capsules 250 mg
Disp: 40
Sig: Open a capsule in 5 mL of water to dissolve; rinse for 1 minute then expectorate 4 times per day

Plus

Rx: Fluocinonide (or clobetasol) ointment 0.05% to be mixed 50/50 with 20% benzocaine paste
Disp: 30 gm
Sig: After completion of each tetracycline rinse, apply to ulcers

Ulcerations NOS (not otherwise specified)/Necrotizing ulcerative stomatitis

Case definition: Large (> 0.5 cm and sometimes up to 3 cm) ulceration(s) with white/yellow necrotic base that may be located on either keratinized or non-keratinized mucosa (note: clinical appearance is similar to that of major aphthous ulcer, but there is no history of recurrent lesions). Necrotizing ulcerative stomatitis presents as localized, painful ulceronecrotic lesions of the oral mucosa that exposes underlying bone or penetrates or extends into contiguous tissues (Figure 6-8). These lesions may extend from areas of necrotizing ulcerative periodontitis. Severe pain may be a prominent feature. These ulcers may be long-standing.

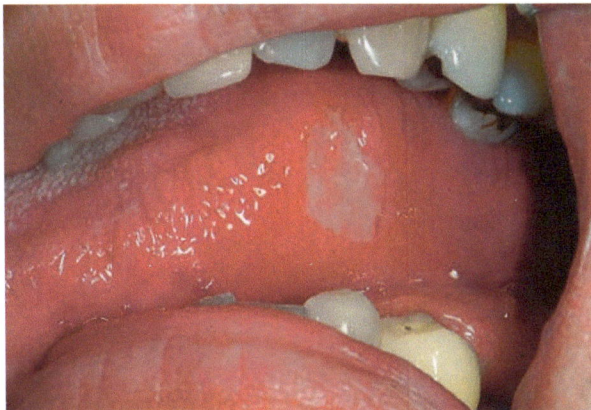

FIGURE 6-8: *Ulceration not otherwise specified (UNOS), left lateral tongue*

Management: A biopsy is necessary to rule out malignancy or etiologies like cytomegalovirus or histoplasmosis, or other deep fungal infections. Once the diagnosis has been confirmed, the treatment is similar to that of major aphthous ulcers.

BACTERIAL INFECTIONS

Necrotizing ulcerative gingivitis (NUG) or necrotizing ulcerative periodontitis (NUP)

Case definition: Presents as destruction of one or more interdental gingival papillae. In the acute stage of the process ulceration, necrosis, and sloughing may be seen with ready hemorrhage and characteristic fetid odor. In the case of necrotizing ulcerative periodontitis, the condition is characterized by soft tissue loss as a result of ulceration or necrosis with exposure, destruction or sequestration of alveolar bone. The teeth may become loosened (Figure 6-9).

Moderate to severe pain may be a prominent feature.

Usually NUP (or NUG) has a sudden onset and is rapidly worsening.

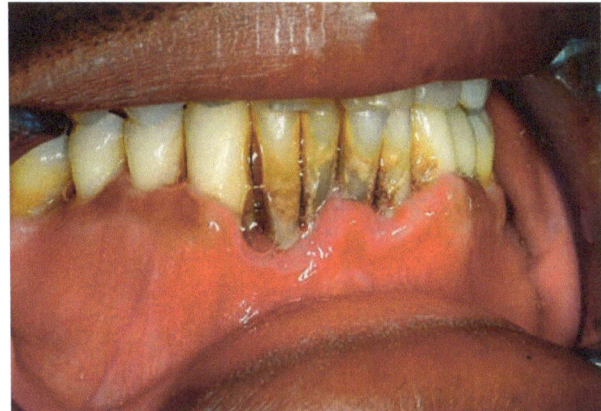

FIGURE 6-9: *Necrotizing ulcerative periodontitis, lower anterior segment*

Management: Under local anesthetic, and using povidone-iodone rinse (with a blunt plastic syringe), affected areas should be debrided and all necrotic soft tissue and bone sequestra removed. The following agents should then be prescribed:

> **Rx**: Metronidazole tabs 250 mg
> Disp: 30
> Sig: Take 2 tabs stat, then 1 tab 4 times per day

If the patient has elevated liver enzymes or cannot avoid alcohol ingestion:

> **Rx**: Amoxicillin Clavulanate tabs 875 mg
> Disp: 20
> Sig: Take 1 tab every 12 hours

Topical antimicrobial rinse:

> **Rx**: Chlorhexidine gluconate 0.12%
> Disp: 16 ounce bottle
> Sig: Rinse with 15 mL for 1 minute and expectorate twice daily

SALIVARY GLAND DISEASE

Parotid enlargement and salivary hypofunction

Case definition: Enlargement of the parotid glands, usually bilateral (Figure 6-10). The condition is usually asymptomatic and long standing. The patient may report a subjective complaint of dry mouth. Salivary hypofunction is usually defined as unstimulated whole salivary flow rate < 0.1 mL/min.

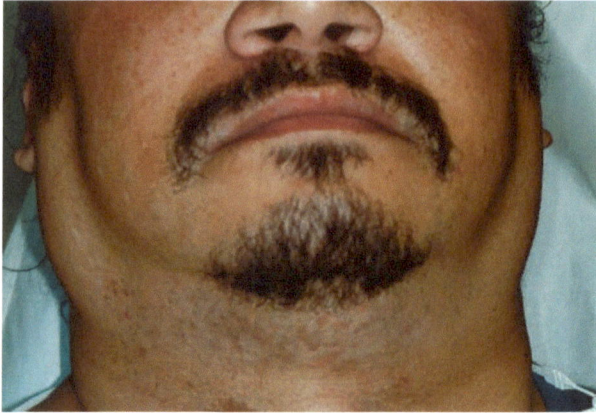

FIGURE 6-10: *Parotid enlargement*

Management: If enlargement is unilateral, or induration is noted upon palpation, it is recommended that the patient be referred to rule out lymphoma. Because of salivary hypofunction, it is important to prevent rampant caries by:

- Prescription of a neutral sodium fluoride 1.1% gel for daily topical application.

- Recommendation to chew sugar-free gum or suck on sugar-free candy to stimulate salivary flow.

- Recommendation to reduce the consumption of products containing caffeine and alcohol.

- Consider cholinergic medication to stimulate salivary function (e.g., pilocarpine tabs 5 mg three times daily; or cevimeline tabs 30 mg three times daily) in consultation with patient's physician.

NEOPLASMS

Oral Kaposi's sarcoma

Case definition: Early lesions are typically flat (or macular) with color ranging from red to purple (Figure 6-11a). At a later stage lesions become nodular, raised and ulcerated (Figure 6-11b). Lesions are predominantly seen on the palate or gingiva. At early stage, lesions are asymptomatic. Mild to moderate pain may develop as lesions become nodular and ulcerated. Local trauma to more advanced lesions may induce bleeding.

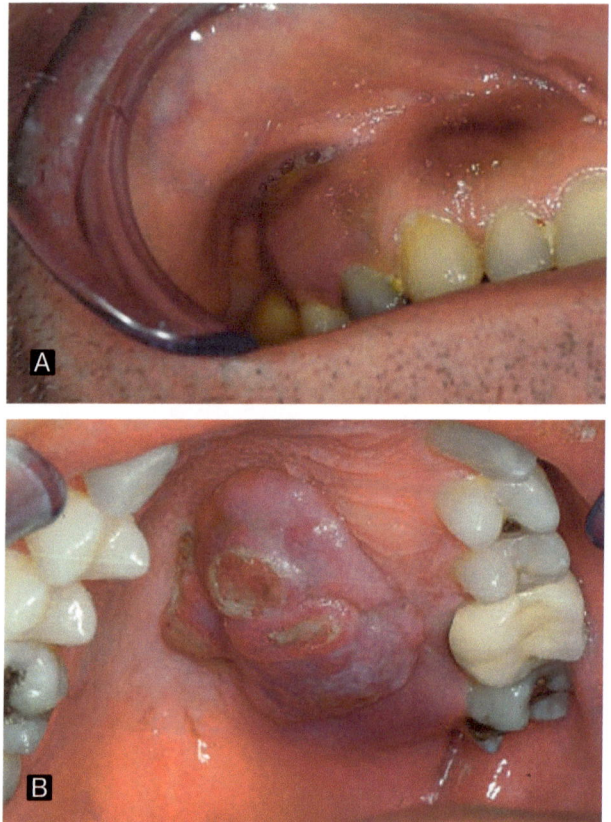

FIGURES 6-11a and 6-11b: *Kaposi sarcoma, gingival (a) and palate (b)*

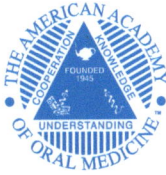

7 HIV Dental Treatment Planning/Modification

Generally there is no justification to modify dental treatment based solely on the patient's HIV status. Treatment planning for HIV-positive patients requires consideration of the patient's present medical status along with prognosis for disease progression and survival. As with any medically complex patient with a potentially fatal, chronic disease, the patient's ability to withstand dental visits, i.e., long or short appointments, as well as changing medical, psychological, and financial resources, will impact dental care delivery. Treatment planning for HIV-positive patients should follow the same order as with other patients: alleviate pain, restore function and attend to aesthetic considerations. This order may have to change with terminally ill patients.

Antibiotic Prophylaxis

HIV-positive patients have demonstrated a higher propensity for developing allergic and adverse reactions to antibiotics during progression of the disease. Thus, judicious use of antibiotics is recommended (Table 7-1).

Coagulopathy

For patients with a history of increased bleeding tendencies, hemorrhagic prone procedures should be approached conservatively, utilizing the tooth-by-tooth approach (i.e., assessing hemostasis after a single extraction prior to proceeding with additional extractions). Appropriate medical history and physical assessment

TABLE 7-1: CONSIDERATIONS FOR ANTIBIOTIC PROPHYLAXIS		
Indications for antibiotic prophylaxis		**No indication for antibiotic prophylaxis**
According to the guidelines set forth by the American Heart Association.# According to guidelines set forth by the American Academy of Orthopaedic Surgeons.*		Based solely on HIV status.
Neutrophil counts below 500 cells/mm^3 in patients not receiving bactericidal antibiotics.		Based on CD4$^+$ or CD8$^+$ cell counts.
When antibiotic prophylaxis is indicated, preferably bactericidal medications should be used, one hour before dental treatment. Please refer to American Heart Association Guidelines# or American Association of Orthopaedic Surgeons Guidelines˙.		
Bactericidal antibiotics		**Bacteriostatic antibiotics**
Amoxicillin	Ampicillin	Azithromycin (low dose)
Azithromycin (high dose)	Cefadroxil	Clarithromycin (low dose)
Cefazolin	Cephalexin	Clindamycin (low dose)
Clarithromycin (high dose)		Erythromycin
Clindamycin (high dose)	Penicillin	Tetracycline
# Prevention of Infective Endocarditis: Guidelines From the American Heart Association http://circ.ahajournals.org/cgi/reprint/CIRCULATIONAHA.106.183095 * Appropriate Use Criteria For the Management of Patients with Orthopaedic Implants Undergoing Dental Procedures http://www.aaos.org/poiudpauc		

should guide patient management to allow sufficient correction of the hemostatic defect so as to diminish the likelihood of significant postsurgical bleeding. HIV positive patients with underlying hemophilia, severe liver cirrhosis, or severe thrombocytopenia may require pre-surgical medical management and blood product transfusion support. Physician consultation and care coordination is recommended for these patients.

Local anesthetics

Delivery of local anesthetics has not been associated with dissemination of intraoral infections. However, deep block injections should be avoided in patients with a recent history of indications for increased bleeding tendencies, until appropriate medical consultation is obtained to guide care. In such cases, local infiltration or intraligamentary injections should be used.

Preventive oral health care

Maintaining good oral hygiene is important to reduce potential oral complications. Decreased salivary flow increases the incidence of caries. Local factors, including subgingival bacteria or candida, may be partially responsible for the more rapid periodontal disease observed in some HIV positive patients.

Suggested protocol:

Recall appointments every six months. This should be reduced to every three months in the severely immuno-suppressed patient and patients exhibiting oral lesions.

Institution of daily antimicrobial mouth rinses for patients with periodontal disease, and a history of necrotizing ulcerative periodontitis.

Fluoride supplements – topically applied mouth rinses, fluoride varnishes or high fluoride concentration tooth-pastes are indicated for patients with decreased salivary flow and increased incidence of caries.

Periodontal therapy

Scaling, curettage and root planing may cause iatrogenic bacteremia but have not been shown to be associated with a higher incidence of systemic signs and symptoms such as fevers and chills in HIV positive patients. A daily antibacterial mouth rinse prior to and following periodontal therapy may further reduce the incidence of local and systemic side effects.

Restorative procedures

Restorative procedures should be performed according to the standard of care. All treatment options available to the patient should be fully explained, including advantages and disadvantages, prior to starting therapy.

Treatment considerations:

- ability to withstand the length of time required for appointment.
- ability to return for sequential visits.
- durability of restoration.
- financial costs associated with care.

Endodontic therapy

Endodontic therapy has not been associated with a higher incidence of postoperative flare-ups. However, should they occur, these flare-ups are generally mild enough to be managed by non-steroidal anti-inflammatory drugs and antibiotics, when needed. Meticulous instrumentation, including avoiding instrumentation beyond the apex, may further reduce the incidence of postoperative flare-ups.

Surgical procedures

Surgical procedures should be performed in a manner to minimize invasion of pathogens from the oral cavity into the deeper facial planes and spaces.

Extractions

Elimination of gross contamination of teeth prior to extractions and gingival flap procedures decreases the potential for dissemination of pathogens.

Extensive surgical interventions

Screening tests for bleeding tendencies, anemia and leukopenia are appropriate prior to extensive surgical interventions, especially in patients with advanced HIV disease (Table 7-2). Consultation with patient's primary physician is recommended.

TABLE 7-2: SUGGESTED LABORATORY TESTS PRIOR TO EXTENSIVE SURGICAL INTERVENTIONS
Platelet count
Prothrombin time/International normalized ratio (PT/INR)
Partial thromboplastin time (PTT)
Hemoglobin level (HgB)
White blood cell count (WBC) and a differential

A major concern when performing any type of procedure that results in tissue manipulation is the healing potential of the tissue. In surgical procedures such as biopsies, surgical extractions, periodontal surgery, apicoectomies or placement of dental implants, no significant impaired healing or significant increased incidence of dry socket have been documented, even in HIV positive patients with severe immune suppression.

NUTRITION

It is well-established that nutrition and diet impact the integrity of the oral cavity. Likewise, oral health impacts dietary intake and nutritional status. Malnutrition is a common complication associated with progressive HIV disease. Pathogenic mechanisms have been implicated in the wasting process, which plays a significant role in the morbidity and mortality of this disease. Many of the oral manifestations found in HIV positive individuals are painful and contribute to the patient's inability to maintain proper nutritional balance. (See Table 7.3) The dentist should play an integral role in detection of oral conditions that impact nutritional status. In patients with suspected nutritional deficiencies, the dentist should assess the essential components of the digestive process which include the dentition, oral mucosa, salivary flow and characteristics, and cranial nerve function. Since the ideal route for nutritional intake is via the gastrointestinal tract, the ability to determine if an individual can consume food by mouth is the beginning of the nutritional assessment process. Although comprehensive nutritional assessment is not a part of training in general dentistry, the dentist should be able to diagnose the oral manifestations of systemic disease, identify impediments to nutritional intake and screen for risk factors of both nutritional deficiency and excess. The dentist should be familiar with general guidelines for optimal nutritional intake, indications for nutritional supplements, common products to recommend and when to refer to nutrition specialists.

In HIV positive patients, all the aforementioned guidelines are particularly important since the disease process as well as therapeutic regimen impact both nutritional status and the oral cavity. Additionally, HIV positive patients may experience more medication interactions, lack of access to medical services, economic instability, food insecurity and social issues all of which confound the morbidity and mortality of the disease.

TABLE 7-3: NUTRITIONAL IMPLICATIONS OF VIRAL AND FUNGAL LESIONS COMMON IN HIV*	
Oral Manifestation or Lesions	**Nutritional Implications**
Viral	
HSV	Painful eating and swallowing, decreased intake, dehydration
CMV	Painful eating and swallowing, may be prolonged healing, decreased intake, dehydration
VZV	Acute phase may have painful eating and swallowing, decreased intake, dehydration
EBV	Usually none
HHV8	Painful eating and swallowing, decreased intake, dehydration, larger lesions may be traumatized
HPV	May interfere with mastication and alter intake
Fungal	
Pseudomembranous Candidiasis	May have painful eating and swallowing, decreased intake, dehydration
Erythematous Candidiasis	Burning sensation may be exacerbated by food selection
Angular Chelitis	Pain and limited mouth opening may decrease intake
Histoplasmosis	May have pain with eating and decreased intake
HSV = herpes simplex; CMV = cytomegalovirus; VZV = varicella zoster virus; EBV = Epstein-Barr Virus; HHV8 = human herpes virus 8; HPV = human papilloma virus	

*Adapted from Patel and Glick. in *Touger-Decker R., Sirois, D., Mobley, C. (eds). Nutrition and Oral Medicine*, Ottowa, Humana Press, 2005, 225-232.

Furthermore, complex alterations in energy utilization, lipid metabolism, hormonal processes, and immune function impact nutritional status as do malabsorption, diarrhea, and vomiting in HIV positive patients.

The general dentist should know that there are nutrition professionals in medical settings, often a registered dietitian, who specializes in HIV nutritional issues including the assessment, nutritional diagnosis, intervention strategies and monitoring of HIV patients within an evidence-based process known as medical nutrition therapy. This comprehensive approach includes individualized anthropometric, biochemical, clinical, and dietary assessment as well as treatment planning and monitoring. Often the HIV positive patient will already be integrated into a multidisciplinary team and a dentist has ready access to consult with the nutrition specialist. In this case, collaboration between the disciplines is important. The dentist's priorities should be to screen for altered oral intake, diagnose and treat restorative as well as mucosal conditions limiting intake, construct a plan for follow-up, and communicate this information to the primary care team.

Nutritional screening tools for use in dental practices are available. Quantifying food intake by recall interviews is another approach used in screening assessments and can begin the dialog with patients for making suggested modifications to increase oral intake.

Inadequate calories and protein are the most immediate concern and are a risk factor for increased mortality in HIV positive patients. Importantly, if an individual does not consume adequate calories, any protein sources will be used as an inefficient source of calories rather than for building tissue. For this reason, caloric intake is the priority for goal setting. While concerns for specific nutrients have been described, it has been difficult to discern the effects of dietary inadequacies of individual nutrients from those of generalized malnutrition. Another reason for caution with supplementation of individual nutrients is the potential interaction with the high number of medications taken by HIV positive patients as well as the potential for toxicity due to the metabolic derangements.

If, however, the general dentist treating HIV positive patients does not have access to a specialty team, then advanced practice skills need to be developed. Comprehensive nutrition assessment and treatment planning is not usually considered the focus of the dentist. The priorities continue to be screening for

nutritional risk through identification of oral factors affecting eating ability. One approach describes common oral lesions in HIV positive patients along with nutritional implications. A best practice would include both prevention and intervention aspects by combining a nutritional screening tool with diagnosis of existing conditions as well as anticipating the presentation of lesions based on other clinical or laboratory indicators.

Nutritional Interventions

Due to the multi-system involvement of HIV and various oral manifestations, nutritional care plans should be individualized. However, if overall oral intake is decreased then often the focus is on high-calorie, high protein, nutrient dense foods which are carefully selected to avoid aggravating existing conditions. Ideally, the priority is to use foods familiar to the patient which are then modified to increase nutritional value and accommodate disease manifestations. The factors responsible for decreased oral intake should be considered in food selection and meal planning. For example, painful or easily traumatized oral lesions require an alteration in food texture to prevent mucosal trauma. Fatigue, anorexia or early satiety may indicate a need to try smaller portions, more frequent meals and nutrient dense snacks. If more calories are needed then commercial nutritional products (Boost®, Ensure®, Instant Breakfast®, etc) can be used to supplement the existing diet. As the needs of the patient change, so must the nutritional care plan. For example, a change in disease status or medications could contribute to oral mucosal changes, altered taste , malabsorption syndromes, nausea or diarrhea, all of which impact food selection, meal planning and may indicate the need for the more targeted nutritional interventions.

Nutrition screening tools

Most medical centers have a clinical nutrition service with screening tools designed to trigger a complete medical nutrition assessment if nutritional risk criteria are met. For HIV, the questions usually focus on the following:

- Weight history including weight change over a specified time period.
- Current diagnoses and co-morbidities.
- Symptoms impacting nutritional status.
- Pertinent labs.

The HIV/AIDS Patient Nutritional Risk Screen developed by the American Dietetic Association for Registered Dieticians providing Medical Nutrition Therapy is included as Table 7-4.

TABLE 7-4: HIV / AIDS PATIENT NUTRITIONAL RISK SCREENING FORM		
Patient Name		
Patient Record Number		
Nutrition Prescription		
Height and Weight History (write numbers next to each item)	Height:	Recent weight lost:
	Weight:	Lowest weight:
	Usual weight:	Highest weight
	Date of HIV Diagnosis (years infected):	
Current Diagnoses (circle all that apply)	Opportunistic infection (e.g., Pneumocystis carinii pneumonia, mycobacterium avium complex)	
	Liver disease (Hepatitis C, B or fatty liver type conditions)	Gastrointestinal disorder (e.g., chronic diarrhea)
	Wasting or weight loss	Lipodystrophy
	Oral thrush	Cancer
	Anemia	Hyperlipidemia
	Diabetes	Renal disease
	Osteoporosis	Tuberculosis
	Other (specify)	
Symptoms (circle all that apply)	Diarrhea	Nausea/vomiting
	Anorexia	Body shape changes: fat atrophy, fat accumulation
	Other (specify)	
Pertinent Labs (write numbers next to each item)	Viral load (current, nadir, highest):	
	CD4 cell count (current, nadir, highest):	
	*Total cholesterol:	*Low-density lipoprotein cholesterol:
	*High-density lipoprotein cholesterol:	*Triglycerides:
	*Glucose:	*Insulin:
	Albumin:	Hemoglobin/hematocrit:
	Testosterone (if male):	
***Fasting, if possible**		

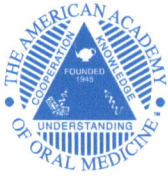

8 Hepatitis (A-E) Pathogenesis and Routes of Transmisison

Hepatitis is defined as an inflammation of the liver in which diffuse or patchy necrosis causes damage to the acini, the functional unit of the liver, resulting in destruction of the liver. Most hepatitis is of viral origin, and several types of viral hepatitis have been identified, including hepatitis A, B, C, D, E viruses. The various hepatitis viruses have different routes of transmission, including enteral (fecal/oral route, also known as lateral when spread person-to-person), parenteral (injection), sexual (exchange of body fluids), and perinatal (from mother to developing fetus, also known as vertical). This monograph will focus on hepatitis A through E.

TRANSMISSION AND PATHOGENESIS

Hepatitis A
Hepatitis A virus (HAV) is transmitted by the fecal/oral route, either person-to-person or by ingestion of contaminated food or water. Common sources of contamination include wells or water supplies and raw or undercooked shellfish from contaminated waters. Poor hygiene, crowded living conditions, travel to areas of the world with poor hygienic conditions and intimate contact may increase the risk of transmission. The incubation period of HAV is from 15 to 45 days. Hepatitis A is a common disease that tends to be of mild severity and is self-limiting. Patients can be assumed to be no longer infectious once 3 weeks have elapsed since the onset of clinical illness. HAV may be prevented by administration of the HAV immune globulin vaccine.

Hepatitis B
Hepatitis B virus (HBV) is a highly infectious blood-borne pathogen capable of being transmitted through exchange of body fluids. In dentistry, it may be transmitted by blood and saliva. The incubation period ranges from 45 to 180 days. Only about 20% of patients exhibit clinical symptoms, which when present usually subside in 2 to 4 weeks. Acute HBV infection in the U. S. occurs principally in adults who have acquired the virus through sexual contact or injection drug use (IDU). High risk groups for HBV are health care workers with frequent exposure to blood, infants born to infected mothers, individuals born in countries endemic for HBV, intravenous drug users, hemodialysis patients, household and sexual contacts of HBV carriers, institutionalized populations, and recipients of infected organs and plasma-derived products. HBV has an acute and chronic state. Approximately 5% of acute infections progress to the chronic state. The younger the individual is when he or she becomes infected with HBV, the higher the carrier state and the more serious the sequelae. HBV infection is a recognized cause of hepatocellular carcinoma (HCC) and may also put individuals at increased risk of developing other cancers, such as non-Hodgkin lymphoma. HBV vaccination has been a highly effective measure to prevent HBV infection and its consequences.

Hepatitis C
Hepatitis C virus (HCV) is a blood-borne virus with an incubation period ranging from 15 to 90 days and a mortality rate of approximately 1-2%. High risk groups for HCV include the following: intravenous drug abusers, hemodialysis patients, health care workers with exposure to blood, and recipients of organs and plasma-derived products. HCV is transmitted primarily through blood; perinatal, sexual and lateral transmission of HCV from infected individuals is low. HCV RNA has also been detected in the saliva of approximately 50% of patients with acute and chronic HCV, and the prevalence of HCV RNA in saliva correlates with HCV viremia. However, in many cases the means of exposure and transmission remains unknown.

HCV has an acute and chronic state. Approximately 20 to 30% of acutely infected individuals exhibit symptoms, and 80% of new infections progress on to chronic infection. With acute HCV, individuals may spontaneously clear the virus. Chronic HCV is a slow, insidious disease, progressing without signs or symptoms for the first two decades after infection until patients have advanced liver disease. Approximately 80% of chronic cases are stable, having mild to moderate histologic disease. The other 20% develop cirrhosis after 20 to 30 years following infection. In patients with cirrhosis, 75% progress slowly, with 1% to 5% developing HCC approximately 30 years following infection. HCV infection also may put individuals at increased risk of developing non-Hodgkin lymphoma and other cancers. Vaccination against HCV is not available at this time.

Hepatitis D
Hepatitis D virus (HDV) requires the existence of the HBV envelope protein for viral replication and pathogenesis. It can be transmitted simultaneously with acute HBV (coinfection) or can infect an individual with an existing HBV infection (superinfection). HDV is transmitted parenterally, sexually, and through the transmucosal exchange of body fluids. In the United States, the most common route of transmission is through intravenous drug use. The incubation period of HDV is from 3 to 13 weeks, and it occurs as an acute and chronic disease. When HDV appears as a coinfection with HBV, it becomes chronic at a rate of <5%. In superinfections, the HDV chronicity rate is 70 to 90%, causing cirrhosis with severe and fulminant disease in up to 70% of the cases. Vaccination for HDV is not available.

Hepatitis E
Hepatitis E virus (HEV) is transmitted enterically via the fecal/oral route. It is primarily seen as a waterborne epidemic in developing countries but may also occur sporadically. The incubation period is usually 3 to 6 weeks and occurs primarily in middle-aged and elderly men. The mortality rate is approximately 1 to 2%; however, in pregnant females, it can be as high as 20%. Groups at risk for the acquisition of HEV include people having close personal contact with infected individuals, people traveling in endemic areas of the world, and those who consume contaminated food or water. Parenteral and lateral transmissions of HEV are rare. The clinical course of hepatitis E infection resembles that of hepatitis A. At present there is no commercially available vaccine for the prevention of hepatitis E. However recent studies have demonstrated the safety and effectiveness of a novel vaccine. Furthermore, the use of this new vaccine when it becomes commercially available may reduce the sporadic and epidemic variants of hepatitis E in endemic areas.

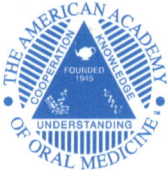

9 Hepatitis (A-E) Epidemiology And Trends

Hepatitis A

Since the introduction of a vaccine against Hepatitis A in 1995 the rates of hepatitis A in the U.S. have steadily declined. The CDC reported 1,390 new cases of HAV in the U.S in 2015.

Hepatitis B

HBV is the most frequent cause of chronic hepatitis. The World Health Organization (WHO) estimates there are 257 million people with chronic HBV worldwide. The highest carrier rates are in Southeast Asia, China, and sub-Saharan Africa. The number of chronic carriers of HBV in the U. S. is estimated between 850,000 and 2.2 million persons. With the introduction of the HBV vaccine in 1982, the number of new HBV infections in the U. S. decreased dramatically from approximately 232,000 to 19,000 cases annually. Age at the time of initial HBV infection is the major determinant of chronicity and impacts the risk of HCC. As many as 90% of infected neonates, 25%-50% of infected children age 1-5 years, and 5% of adults infected with acute HBV develop chronic infection. Approximately 25% of HBV carriers who became infected during childhood and 15% of HBV carries who became infected during after childhood develop progressive disease that often leads to complications such as cirrhosis or HCC. Vaccination against HBV, as well as standard infection control precautions has significantly reduced the risk of dental healthcare workers acquiring HBV. Historically dental health care workers had a higher risk of HBV infection that was 3 to 5 times higher than the general population.

Hepatitis C

In the U. S., an estimated 2.7-3.9 million people (1.8%) are infected with HCV. Most infections are diagnosed in middle-aged adults with injection drug use has been the predominant risk factor for HCV infection. In the U. S., 30,000 acute new cases occur annually, with 25% experiencing symptoms, and 19,000 deaths occur annually from cirrhosis and HCC. The incidence of HCV has declined significantly since the late 1980s with the introduction of a highly sensitive HCV test to prevent transfusion of contaminated blood products. There are six distinct HCV genotypes (genotypes 1–6) and more than 50 subtypes. Genotype 1 is the most common HCV genotype in the United States. Treatment of HCV

Hepatitis D

HDV is more prevalent in persons of lower socioeconomic status in Africa and South America, Turkey, Mongolia, southern Italy, and the Soviet Union. In the U. S. HDV accounts for less than 5% of the cases of chronic hepatitis. HDV and HBV coinfection is almost exclusively observed in IDU's in the U.S. Superinfection of HDV on chronic HBV accelerates the progression to cirrhosis.

Hepatitis E

HEV is the U.S. is rare but it is more common in the developing world where clean water and environmental sanitation contribute to its prevalence. Reported cases of HEV in the U.S. have been isolated and consisting of people who recently traveled to endemic regions. HEV occurs sporadically or in epidemics in parts of India, Asia, Mexico, and North and West Africa. It is not a significant problem in the U.S.

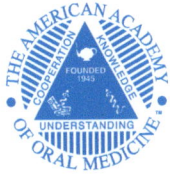

10   Hepatitis (A-E) Clinical Disease Course

Acute viral hepatitis (defined as infection of 6 months or less) is characterized by virus replication in hepatocytes, inflammation, degeneration, and necrosis of liver cells. As a result, the damaged liver inefficiently conjugates bilirubin, a degradation product of hemoglobin, and bilirubin accumulates in the blood, is deposited in the tissues and excreted in the urine. When bilirubin accumulates in the plasma, icterus (jaundice) occurs.

During a nonspecific viral prodrome phase, symptoms may include fatigue, weakness, anorexia, nausea and vomiting, fever, diarrhea, headache, abdominal pain, and myalgias. This is followed by the icteric phase, in which develop- ment of jaundice and elevated liver enzyme levels occur. Icterus occurs in approximately 70% of HAV cases, 30% of HBV, and 25% of HCV and HEV. Most cases of HAV and HEV resolve without complications. Acute HBV, HCV and HDV may persist and replicate in the liver, causing a carrier state (chronic infection).

A serious complication of acute viral hepatitis is fulminant hepatitis (acute liver failure), which is characterized by massive hepatocellular destruction, jaundice, remarkably high levels of serum aminotransferases and a mortality rate of approximately 80%. Fulminant hepatitis occurs most commonly in individuals coinfected or superinfected with HBV and HDV.

Chronic hepatitis is characterized by persistence of low levels of virus in the liver and serum viral antigens for longer than six months without signs of liver disease. It is defined as hepatitis inflammation, necrosis, and fibrosis and is often asymptomatic for 20 to 30 years. The chronic hepatitis carrier state may persist for decades or may cause liver disease by progressing to chronic active hepatitis, characterized by active virus replication in the liver, virus levels in the serum, persistent necrosis, and elevated liver enzymes for more than 6 months. The massive destruction of liver tissue can result in cirrhosis, HCC, liver failure and, ultimately, death. Approximately 5% of patients infected with HBV, 25% of HBV carriers, and 40 to 50% of those infected with HCV develop chronic active hepatitis. Chronic liver destruction and fibrosis lead to cirrhosis in approximately 20% of chronic hepatitis cases. Approximately 1 to 5% of these patients develop HCC. Liver transplantation is the only treatment option for patients with end-stage liver cirrhosis.

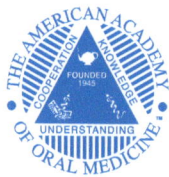

11 Hepatitis (A-E) Medications and Implications for Dentistry

Supportive care is the only measure currently available for acute hepatitis. It is recommended that patients with intractable vomiting, dehydration, electrolyte imbalances, older than 50 years or are immunocompromised should be admitted to a hospital. Patients with acute hepatitis should be reminded to avoid hepatotoxic agents such as acetaminophen or alcohol. Viral antigen and alanine aminotransferase levels should be monitored for 6 months so that it can be determined whether the hepatitis is resolving. Lamivudine, adefovir dipivoxil, and other antiviral therapies may improve clinical response in severe cases of acute HBV infection and reduce morbidity and mortality in chronic HBV.

Chronic hepatitis infection may be progressive and, therefore, requires management. Antiviral treatment is indicated for patients with elevated aminotransferase levels, clinical or biopsy evidence of progressive disease, or both. Therapeutic options for HBV includes the addition of oral nucleoside/nucleotide analogs. In the U.S. lamivudine,

telbivudine, entecavir, adefovir, tenofovir, and peg-IFN-2a are approved for the treatment of adults with chronic HBV. Lamivudine, entecavir, adefovir, tenofovir, and peg-IFN-2b approved for the treatment of children with chronic HBV. Approximately one-third of patients chronically infected with HBV and 20% of patients with HCV and 15% with HDV have a sustained response to therapy. Generally the side effects of treatment are infrequent and treatment is safe. Adverse effects can include flu-like symptoms, cytopenia, anorexia and weight loss, pancreatitis, myopathy, and acute renal failure.

Due to the potential adverse effects of medications, a complete blood count and differential is recommended prior to surgical and sedation procedures for patients taking nucleoside/nucleotide analogs. See Table 11-1 for medications used in the management of chronic hepatitis, adverse reactions, dental implications and oral manifestations of these medications.

TABLE 11-1: MEDICATIONS USED FOR MANAGEMENT OF HEPATITIS AND SIDE EFFECTS		
Type of Hepatitis	**Medication**	**Potential Side Effects**
Hepatitis B and C	Interferon α-2a or α-2b	Bone marrow suppression, fatigue, myalgia, arthralgia, headache, depression, malaise, tachycardia, alopecia, cardiac or renal failure; autoimmune disorders: interstitial pneumonia, systemic lupus erythematosus, autoimmune hemolytic anemia, hypothyroidism, immune thrombocytopenia, sarcoidosis; mucositis, ulcerative stomatitis, glossitis, dysgeusia, xerostomia
Hepatitis B	Lamivudine	Headache, fatigue, insomnia, nausea, diarrhea, pancreatitis, abdominal pain, vomiting, neutropenia, myalgia, neuropathy, musculoskeletal pain, dizziness, depression, thrombocytopenia, mucositis, ulcerative stomatitis
	Adefovir dipivoxil	Increase in serum creatinine, headache, abdominal pain, diarrhea, malaise, nausea
	Entecavir	Headache, fatigue, dizziness, hyperglycemia, diarrhea, nausea, increased creatinine, alopecia
	Telbivudine	Fatigue, headache, myalgia, arthralgia, dizziness, insomnia, diarrhea, nausea, neutropenia, neuropathy, thrombocytopenia
Hepatitis C	Ribavirin	Hemolytic anemia, teratogenicity, fatigue, headache, fever, insomnia, depression, dizziness, impaired concentration, alopecia, nausea, vomiting, diarrhea, leukopenia, anemia, myalgia, arthralgia, xerostomia, dysgeusia; aplastic anemia, autoimmune disorders

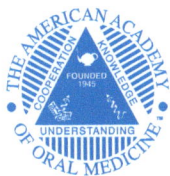

12 Hepatitis (A-E) Pertinent Laboratory Tests

Serum antigen and antibody tests are available for hepatitis types A through E. These serological tests are required for identifying the viral agent and for distinguishing acute, resolved and chronic infection or immunity against hepatitis viruses (Table 12-1 on following page). Screening for HCV, HDV and HEV are performed with enzyme immunoassays.

Serum transaminase levels become elevated as the result of damage to infected liver cells. Aspartate aminotransferase (AST) and alanine aminotransferase (ALT) are sensitive indicators of liver injury and acute viral hepatitis and reflect the degree of hepatocellular damage. ALT is a more specific indicator than is AST for detecting acute and chronic hepatitis. Patients are diagnosed as having mild elevations when liver function test levels are less than three times the normal levels; moderate elevations when values range from 3 to 20 times higher than normal, and severe elevations when values are greater than 20-fold higher.

Another blood test useful in the diagnosis of hepatitis is serum bilirubin, which reflects a balance between the degradation of hemoglobin and its hepatic elimination. Normal serum bilirubin levels are <1.1 mg/dL, and clinical jaundice is associated with levels of 2 to 3 mg/dL. The serum alkaline phosphatase level may be mildly elevated or normal; however, this is a relatively nonspecific test.

More severe disease diminishes the liver's ability to produce coagulation factors, resulting in persistent elevations in the prothrombin time (PT), partial thromboplastin time (PTT) and abnormal hemostasis. PT is a universal indicator of liver failure. Patients can safely be treated when PT falls within the normal range and a platelet count is above 50,000/mL. Serum albumin may also be decreased in severe forms of chronic hepatitis, indicating that hepatic synthetic function is impaired. See Table 12-2 (on following page) for blood tests used as indicators of liver dysfunction.

Histological examination of hepatic tissue is used to assess and grade the level of fibrosis and cirrhosis and help guide treatment options. Although the liver biopsy is considered the standard of care there are issues associated with this invasive procedure. Major complications may include bleeding, hemobilia, bile peritonitis, bacteremia, sepsis, pneumothorax, hemothorax and death. More recently physicians are using indirect laboratory testing to ascertain hepatic fibrosis and cirrhosis in hepatitis C patients. There are three validated commercial serum marker systems available in the U.S to assess hepatic fibrosis. They are: FibroTest/FibroSure (LabCorp), Hepascore (Quest Diagnostics), and FibroSpect (Prometheus Corp). The aspartate aminotransferase to platelet ratio (APRI) calculated using routine laboratory tests data is also used. All these tests can distinguish patients with significant fibrosis but are unable to differentiate between the stages of fibrosis.

Viral Agent	Viral marker	Initial Antibody Response	Antibody Immunity Response	Transmission	Vaccine
HAV		IgM anti-HAV (current or recent infection)	IgG anti-HAV	Fecal-oral	Yes
HBV	HBsAg (surface antigen-1st response, acute infection) HBeAg (envelope antigen-chronic infection) HBcAg (core antigen) HBV DNA	IgM anti-HBc IgG anti-HBc anti-HBeAg anti-HBsAg	anti-HBs anti-HBe	Parenteral, sexual, perinatal	Yes
HCV	HCV RNA	anti-HCV		Parenteral, sexual? perinatal?	No
HDV	HDV RNA	IgM anti-HDV IgG anti-HDV		Parenteral, sexual, perinatal	No
HEV	HEV RNA	IgM anti-HEV IgG anti-HEV		Fecal-oral	Under development

TABLE 12-1: SERUM ANTIGEN AND ANTIBODY TESTS FOR HEPATITIS A THROUGH E

TABLE 12-2: BLOOD TESTS THAT ARE USEFUL IN PATIENTS WITH LIVER DYSFUNCTION

Test	Normal Range	Abnormal	Implications of abnormal test
Serum Bilirubin	<0.3-1.0 mg/dL	≥ 2.5 mg/dL (jaundice)	Liver dysfunction
ALT	Males: 10-40 U/L Females: 7-35 U/L	Mild: < 3x higher than normal Moderate: 3-20x higher than normal Severe: >20x higher than normal	Liver dysfunction More sensitive than AST in the detection of acute and chronic hepatitis
AST	Males: 14-20 U/L Females: 10-36 U/L	Elevations of 10-100 x normal	Liver dysfunction Less sensitive than ALT in the detection of acute and chronic hepatitis
Alkaline phosphatase	25-100 U/L	Elevated, correlated with elevated AST, ALT	Liver dysfunction; impaired ability to excrete alkaline phosphatase
Serum albumin	35-48 g/L	<35 g/L	Chronic liver disease, cirrhosis
PT	10-12 seconds	> 20 seconds	Prolonged bleeding with surgical procedures
INR	1.0-3.5 seconds	≥ 3.5 sec	Prolonged bleeding with surgical procedures
PTT	21-35 seconds	>35 seconds	Prolonged bleeding with surgical procedures >70 seconds: spontaneous bleeding
Platelet count	140,000-400,000/mL	<50,000/mL	Coagulopathy: prolonged bleeding with surgical procedures; decreased ability or inability to form a blood clot <20,000/mL: tendency for spontaneous bleeding

ALT= alanine aminotransferase, AST= aspartate aminotransferase, PT= prothrombin time, INR= international normalized ratio, PTT= partial thromboplastin time

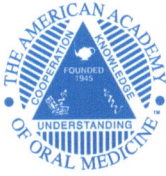

13 Hepatitis (A-E) Common Oral Manifestations and Management

In patients with acute hepatitis, during the icterus phase, jaundice can be seen in the oral mucosa (see Figures 14a and 14b on the following page). Jaundice is best visualized in the immovable and movable soft palate, the floor of the mouth along the lingual frenum, and the buccal mucosa. Viral-induced liver disease can cause gingival bleeding, petechiae, and ecchymoses. Hepatitis B and C viruses are present in whole saliva of infected humans, and HCV in saliva may lead to lymphocytic sialadenitis in selected patients.

Patients with chronic HCV may present with extrahepatic manifestations considered to be of autoimmune origin, such as thrombocytopenic purpura, keratoconjunctivitis sicca, vasculitis, lichen planus, and Sjögren-like syndrome. Lichen planus associated with chronic HCV can be intraoral or extraoral and appears in about 5 to 10% of patients with chronic HCV, with higher prevalence in Italy and Japan than in North America. Patients affected with Sjögren-like syndrome often have keratoconjunctivitis sicca (dry eyes), and clinical abnormalities of oral dryness and abnormal sialography are variable. Also, interferon used in the management of chronic hepatitis may cause various autoimmune disorders that may have oral manifestations, such as systemic lupus erythematosus and recurrent sarcoidosis with or without bilateral swelling of parotid glands.

Metastases of HCC to the orofacial complex are rare. Generally, they appear as rapidly expanding, vascular, and hemorrhagic masses located posterior to the premolar region and extending into the mandibular ramus.

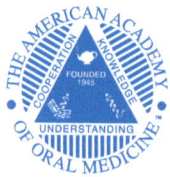

14 Hepatitis (A-E) Dental Treatment Planning/ Modification

Patients with Active Hepatitis

Only urgent care treatment should be administered on a patient with active hepatitis. Urgent care should be provided in an isolated operatory with adherence to strict standard precautions and aerosols should be minimized. Drugs metabolized in the liver should be avoided as much as possible. If surgical intervention is warranted, coagulopathy is a concern due to failure to synthesize prothrombin as well as other clotting factors. Consequently, a pre-operative platelet count PT/INR and PTT should be obtained.

Patients with a History of Hepatitis

Patients with a known history of HBV and HCV should be evaluated to determine carrier status, activity of disease, and liver function. In patients who are carriers, dental treatment may have to be modified if moderate-to-severe liver disease is present. Elevations of serum transaminases indicate risk for altered drug metabolism, and numerous drugs commonly prescribed by dentists are primarily metabolized in the liver. Consultation with the patient's physician is recommended, as such drugs may be able to be used in reduced amounts and administered at increased intervals. For example, most amide local anesthetics are metabolized in the liver and may reach toxic levels with lower doses. Some antibiotics (erythromycin, metronidazole, tetracyclines) should be avoided completely; acetaminophen should be avoided, while nonsteroidal anti-inflammatory agents should be used cautiously due to an increased risk of gastrointestinal bleeding and interference with fluid balance. Further, caution should be used with prescribing certain sedatives (diazepam, barbiturates), and some sulfonamides. Severe liver disease (i.e., cirrhosis) increases the risk for infection, and peri-operative antibiotics may be indicated for extractions and surgical procedures.

FIGURES 14a and 14b:
Note the jaundice of the skin and scleral icterus (a) and the mucosal icterus in this patient with hepatitis C associated cirrhosis (b)

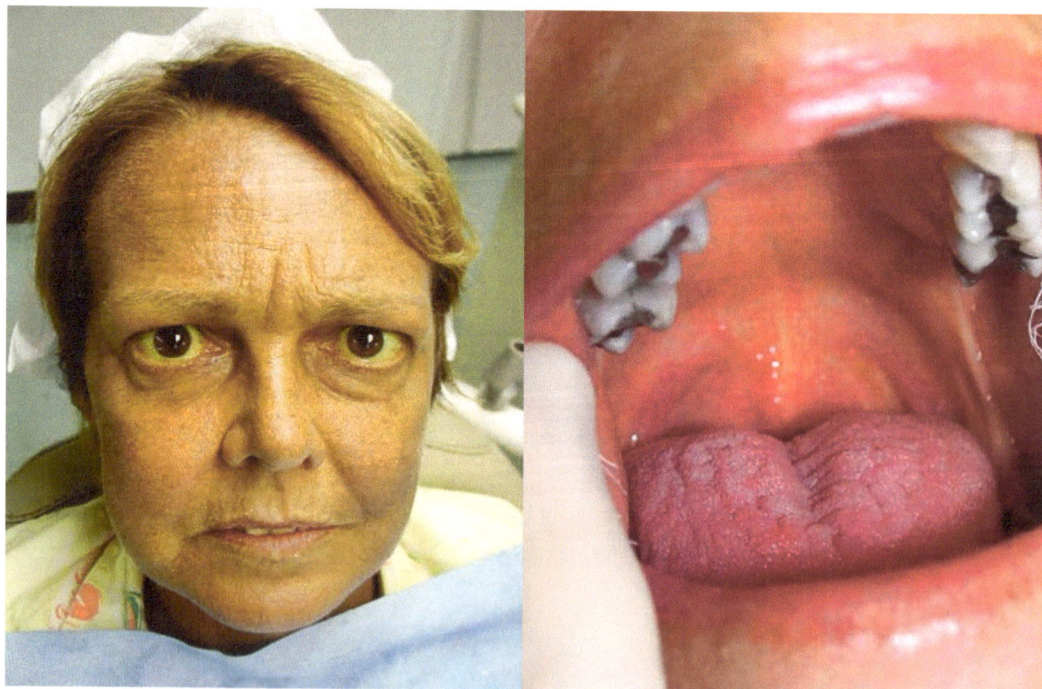

A concern for proper hemostasis is a significant risk in people with liver disease. In chronic hepatitis and cirrhosis, prolonged bleeding after surgical procedures is commensurate with the degree of hepatocyte destruction and can be assessed by ordering a PT/ INR and PTT. When INR values are between 1.0 and 3.5, it is usually considered safe to perform surgical procedures as long as the other measures of hemostasis are normal and local hemostatic measures (gel foam, topical thrombin, pressure dressings, and soft diet) are employed. Platelet counts should also be assessed. Counts above 50,000/mm^3 are generally considered safe when conservative surgical technique is employed and other measures of hemostasis are within the normal reference range. In patients with severe liver disease, there may be elevated PT/INR, PTT and significantly reduced platelet counts that taken together significantly reduce the patient's capacity for obtaining effective hemostasis after dental surgical procedures. Advanced oral surgical procedures or any dental procedures with the potential to cause bleeding due to coagulopathy may need to be provided in a hospital setting.

Liver transplantation is a potential life-saving approach for patients with end-stage chronic hepatitis. The pre- and post-transplant patient may be at increased risk for infection due to immunosuppressant therapy.

Post-exposure protocol

In situations of known exposure, the CDC recommendation for post-exposure prophylaxis is dependent on the type of virus suspected or known, and whether the exposure is from a person with acute or chronic disease. Firstly, all health care workers with potential exposure to blood and body fluids should receive the full series of HBV vaccinations. If a dental health care worker is exposed (percutaneous exposure by a sharp or needlestick) to the blood or bodily fluid of an HBsAg-positive person, antibody titers should be tested. If the individual's titer levels are inadequate, hepatitis B immune globulin is to be given within 24 hours and the vaccine (booster if previously vaccinated, initiate vaccination if unvaccinated) within 14 days. For those with successful vaccination the need for booster is not well documented, although the titer in the serum may decrease slowly and past recommendations have included a booster vaccination ten years following primary immunization. The risk that a dental health care worker will contract HBV from HBV carriers through a sharps injury may be as high as 30% if the provider has not been vaccinated or did not obtain an antibody response following immunization. If titer levels are adequate, no further action is required.

The risk that a dental health care worker will contract HCV from HCV carriers through a sharps injury is approximately 1.8%. The CDC does not currently recommend post-exposure prophylaxis for HCV as there is no evidence of effective agents for this purpose. The CDC current guidelines recommend: a) the source person be baseline, b) the person exposed be baseline tested for HCV antibodies no later than 48 hours post exposure, positive results would be immediately tested for HCV RNA c) individuals with negative antibodies to HCV or positive to HCV RNA should be retested for HCV RNA at 3 weeks, and d) individuals responding positive to HCV RNA testing should be referred for further care.

Further information can be found at: https://www.cdc.gov/hepatitis/pdfs/testing-followup-exposed-hc-personnel.pdf

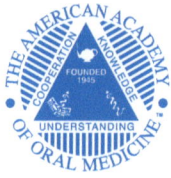

15 Tuberculosis Pathogenesis and Routes of Transmission

Tuberculosis (TB) is one of the world's most widespread and deadly infections. *M. tuberculosis*, the organism that causes tuberculosis infection and disease, infects an estimated 20 to 40% of the world's population. Infection with *M. tuberculosis* begins when a susceptible person inhales airborne droplet nuclei containing viable organisms. Tubercle bacilli that reach the alveoli are ingested by alveolar macrophages. Infection follows if the inoculum escapes alveolar macrophages microbicidal activity. Once the infection is established, lymphatic and hematogenous dissemination of tuberculosis typically occurs before the development of an effective immune response. The interval from infection to development of active TB is widely variable, ranging from a few weeks to decades. Most TB cases result from reactivation of a tubercle; only 5 to 10% of cases result at the time of the initial infection.

The initial stage of the infection is called *primary tuberculosis* and is usually absent of clinical and radiographic signs. In most persons with intact cell-mediated immunity, T cells and macrophages surround the organisms in granulomas that limit their multiplication and spread. Limitation and local containment of the infection may be caused by a variety of factors, including host resistance, host immune capabilities, and virulence of the microorganism. Once the infection has been successfully interrupted and contained, the lesion heals spontaneously, and then undergoes encapsulation and calcification. The infection is contained but not eradicated, since viable organisms may lie dormant within the granulomas for years to decades. Individuals with this *latent tuberculosis* infection do not have active disease and cannot transmit the organism to others. However, reactivation of disease may occur if the host's immune defenses are impaired. Active TB will develop in approximately 10% of individuals with latent TB infection who are not given preventive therapy; half of these cases occur in the 2 years following primary infection. Up to 50% of HIV-infected patients will develop active

TB within 2 years after infection with *M. tuberculosis*.

In approximately 5% of cases, the immune response is inadequate and the host develops *progressive primary tuberculosis*, accompanied by both pulmonary and constitutional symptoms. Approximately 90% of TB in adults represents activation of latent disease.

Successful infection by *M. tuberculosis* depends on the initial encounter between the pathogen and the host cell, usually the macrophage. The surface characteristics of the pathogen and host cell will determine the outcome. Although mycobacteria are gram positive, their wax-rich cell wall confers the unique features and thus they are classified as acid-fast bacilli. The abundant cell wall glycolipids and mycolic acids are responsible for the immune response. *M. tuberculosis* has been proposed to bind to a variety of host cell receptors, including complement receptors, Fc receptors, surfactant protein receptors, CD 14, and the macrophage mannose receptor via a variety of surface molecules. The receptor used to enter the macrophage affects the cellular response. For example, interaction of the *M. tuberculosis* with the Fc receptor induces the production of reactive oxygen permitting phagosome-lysosome fusion. The variety of receptors that could be utilized by *M. tuberculosis* to enter host cells, led researchers to believe that there is no one "preferred route." Once inside the macrophage, *M. tuberculosis* faces the problem of establishing residence inside the primary host effector cell. Mycobacteria have evolved a mechanism to exploit the macrophages as an intracellular host. One of the major problems that the bacteria face is the acquisition of essentials nutrients in the intracellular environment. Macrophages require iron as a cofactor in the induction of the microbicidal effector mechanisms, while bacteria themselves have an obligate requirement for iron for their intracellular survival. There are different methods that *M. tuberculosis* uses to ensure that its iron supply is not limited.

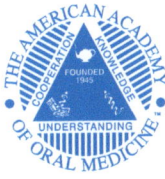

16 Tuberculosis Epidemiology and Trends

Tuberculosis is the ninth leading cause of death worldwide. In the latest report dated 2016, WHO estimates that 10.4 million individuals were living with active TB and further there were 6.3 million new cases diagnosed. Among the 1.67 million persons who died from TB in the year 2016, 1.3 million were HIV seronegative and 374,000 HIV seropositive.

In 2015, a total of 9,557 TB cases were reported in the U. S. For the same period, the case rate of TB among foreign-born persons was 15.1 per 100,000 population; the majority of these cases were among persons living in the United States 5 years or longer. Among U.S.-born persons the TB case rate was 1.2 cases per 100,000 persons. Foreign-born persons and racial/ethnic minorities continue to have TB disproportionate to their respective populations. For example the Tb case rate per 100,000 persons for American natives is 6.1, Asians 18.2, Blacks and African Americans 5.0, Latinos 4.8 and Whites 0.6. Drug-resistant TB is a continuing threat.

The world can be divided into two sections based on the extent of TB epidemics. The low prevalence areas are composed of countries that experienced serious TB epidemics after the 18th century, slowly overcoming them and finally reducing the incidence rate to 100 per 100,000 or less. The high prevalence areas include countries with an incidence rate above 100 per 100,000 that have experienced TB epidemics after the 20th century. The low prevalence countries are industrialized, while the high prevalence countries are mostly developing countries or areas. Interestingly enough, the latter accounts for two-thirds of the world population, and as much as 95% of the estimated number of newly occurring TB patients globally. Also, there are differences in the characteristics of TB. In high prevalence countries, most patients are in their 20s to 40s, resulting in an important socioeconomic loss as this is the most productive generation. In contrast, among low prevalence countries, TB involves the elderly, and high risk groups (HIV, diabetes, immunosuppressed) presenting a challenge to medical services.

As a result of the global efforts in TB control under the Directly Observed Treatment Short-Course (DOTS) strategy since the 1990s, the incidence of TB is estimated to have declined around 2003. Unfortunately in the developing world new challenges in the treatment of TB have emerged. One if these challenges is multi-drug resistant (MDR) TB. In 2016, there were 600 000 new cases of Tb with resistance to rifampicin (RRTB), the most effective first-line treatment drug and 490 000 of these patients had multidrug-resistant TB (MDR-TB). Almost half (47%) of these drug resistant cases of Tb originated in India, China and the Russian Federation.

Another challenging issue is the co-infection of HIV and *M. tuberculosis*. In 2016, 6.3 million new cases of TB were reported and approximately 476,774 were also HIV seropositive. Currently, 10% of active TB patients, estimated at greater than 1 million people, are HIV seropositive. Twenty nine percent of the global TB deaths are co-infected with HIV.

Another challenging issue in TB is children. In 2016, an estimated 1 million children became ill with TB and 250, 000 children died of TB (including children with HIV associated TB).

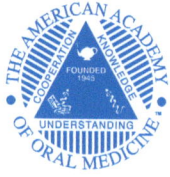

17 Tuberculosis Clinical Disease Course

Primary infection with *M. tuberculosis* in about 90% of patients results in few manifestations other than a positive tuberculin test and radiographic findings. The patient with pulmonary TB typically presents with slowly progressive constitutional symptoms of malaise, anorexia, weight loss, fever, and night sweats. Chronic cough is the most common pulmonary symptom. The cough may be dry at first but typically becomes productive of sputum as the disease progresses. Dyspnea is unusual unless there is extensive disease. Manifestations of extrapulmonary disease occur in about 10 to 20% of cases, more often in patients co-infected with HIV. These manifestations may include localized lymphadenopathy with the development of sinus tracts, back pain over the affected area of the spine, gastrointestinal disturbances, dysuria and hematuria, and neurological deficit. On physical evaluation the patient appears chronically ill and malnourished.

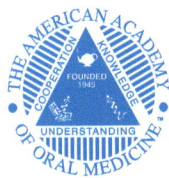

18 Tuberculosis Medications and Implications for Dentistry

Comprehensive treatment of TB requires coordination between clinical care and public health policies. The objectives of therapy are to eliminate all tubercle bacilli from an infected patient while avoiding the emergence of clinically significant drug resistance. The basic principles of anti-tuberculosis treatment are (1) to administer multiple medications to which the organisms are susceptible; (2) to add at least two new anti-tuberculosis agents to a regimen when treatment failure is suspected; (3) to provide the safest, most effective therapy in the shortest period of time; and (4) to ensure adherence of the therapy. All suspected and confirmed cases of TB should be reported to the local health departments. Public health departments will perform case investigations on source and patient contacts to explore if other individuals with untreated, infectious TB are present in the community. Infectious contacts should be treated for latent TB infection. Patients with TB should be treated by physicians who are experienced in the management of TB.

Non-adherence to anti-tuberculosis medications is a major cause of treatment failure, continued transmission of TB, and the development of drug resistance. Adherence to treatment can be improved by providing detailed patient education about TB and its treatment. Directly observed short-course therapy (DOTS), which requires that a health care worker physically observe the patient ingest anti-tuberculosis medications. Observation is done daily or several times per week in the home, medical office, hospital, or other patient convenient location. DOTS improves adherence to the treatment. Most patients with previously untreated pulmonary TB can be effectively treated with either a 6 month or a 9 month regimen. However, the 6-month option is preferred. The initial phase of a 6-month regimen consists of 2 months of daily isoniazid, rifampin, pyrazinamide, and ethambutol. Once the isolate is determined to be isoniazid-sensitive, ethambutol may be discontinued. If the *M. tuberculosis* isolate is susceptible to isoniazid and rifampin, the second phase of the therapy consists of isoniazid and rifampin for a minimum of 4 additional months, with treatment to extend at least 3 months beyond documentation of conversion of sputum cultures to negative for *M. tuberculosis*. Patients who cannot or should not (pregnant women) take pyrazinamide should receive daily isoniazid and rifampin along with ethambutol for 4-8 weeks.

Patients with drug-resistant TB represent a major problem and require careful supervision and management. Tuberculosis resistant only to isoniazid can be treated with a 6-month regimen of rifampin, pyrazinamide, and ethambutol. Multidrug-resistant tuberculosis (MDRTB) requires an individualized daily observed treatment plan under the supervision of a clinician with experience. Treatment regimens are based on the patient's overall status and the results of the susceptibility tests. Most MDRTB isolates are resistant to at least isoniazid and rifampin and require a minimum of three medications to which the organism is susceptible. These regimens are continued until culture conversion is documented.

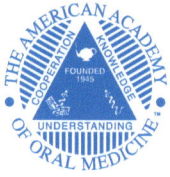

19 Tuberculosis Pertinent Laboratory Tests

Important efforts have been made to accelerate the development and expansion of new diagnostic technologies for TB testing. However, TB case detection still remains dependent upon sputum smear and culture, and radiographic and clinical symptoms. Patients suspected of having active TB usually receive a chest radiograph and serial sputum smears and cultures for AFB (acid-fast bacilli). The chest radiograph is suspicious of tuberculosis when infiltrates (with or without cavity) are noted in the apical-posterior segments of the upper lung and superior segments of the lower lobe. Chest radiographs may be normal in patients with endobronchial disease or HIV disease with active TB. In the sputum smear at least 5,000 to 10,000 organism should be present for a smear to be positive. The more acid-fast bacilli seen, the more infectious the patient is. The sensitivity and specificity of the sputum culture is high (82%, 99% respectively) and it is considered the "gold standard" in the diagnosis of TB. Although several studies have been published regarding the use of interferon-γ release assays incorporating *M. tuberculosis*-specific antigens in the diagnosis of latent TB infection, their value in predicting the progression of latent infection needs to be established.

The tuberculin test identifies individuals who have been infected with *M. tuberculosis* but does not differentiate between active and latent infection. The test is used to evaluate a person who has symptoms of TB, an asymptomatic person who may be infected with *M. tuberculosis*, or to establish the prevalence of TB infection in a population. Routine testing of individuals at low risk for TB is not recommended. The Mantoux test is the preferred method: 0.1 mL of purified protein derivate (PPD) containing 5 tuberculin units is injected intradermally in the dorsal surface of the forearm. The transverse width in millimeters of induration at the skin test site should be measured after 48-72 hours. An area of induration measuring less than 5 mm is considered a negative result. An area of induration measuring greater than 5 mm is considered a positive result if the patient has had close contact with an infectious person or an abnormal chest radiograph consistent with TB, or if she or he is suspected or known to be HIV positive or immunocompromised. An area of induration that measures 10 mm or greater is considered positive if significant risk factors are present. Induration of at least 15 mm is considered positive for everyone.

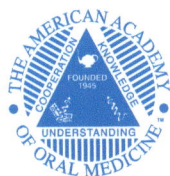

20 Tuberculosis Common Oral Manifestations and Management

Tuberculosis is rare in the oral cavity. Oral lesions can present at any age but are most commonly seen in men about 30 years of age and in children. Oral lesions usually appear secondary to primary TB elsewhere, although primary infection of the oral mucosa by *M. Tuberculosis* has been described. Lesions are found in the posterior part of the mouth, possible related with lymphatic distribution. The clinical presen-tation of the TB lesions of the oral mucosa varies widely, including ulceration, diffuse inflammatory lesions, granulomas and fissures. The tongue is a prevalent site of presentation, but lesions have been noted in the buccal mucosa, gingiva, floor of the mouth, lips, and palate. (Figure 20-1) Tuberculosis lymphadenitis may involve the cervical lymph nodes. Atypical mycobacterium is involved in cervical lymphadenitis in children.

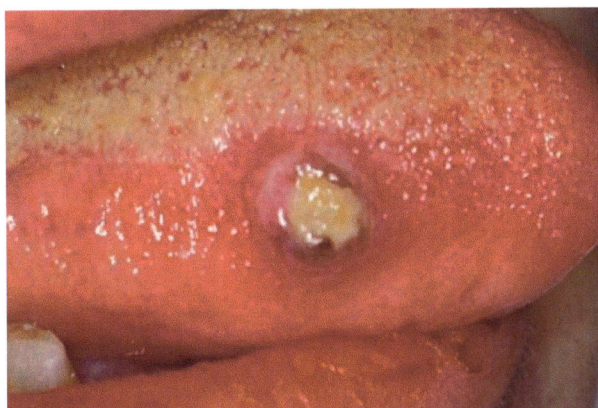

FIGURE 20-1: *Tuberculosis lesion on the lateral border of the tongue*

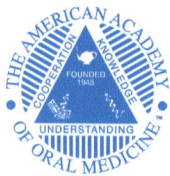

21 Tuberculosis Dental Treatment Planning/ Modification

Tuberculosis has been recognized for many years as an occupational risk for health care workers. However, with the advent of chemotherapy and the reduction in the incidence of the disease in the mid 1980s, awareness of the problem declined. Several studies using tuberculin testing indicates that there has been an increase in *M. Tuberculosis* contact among health care workers.

In the general dental evaluation of patients with TB, it is important to differentiate patients with active TB taking appropriate medications from patients with active TB without treatment, and from those with positive tuberculin test (*M. Tuberculosis* positive but not with active disease). The dentist should question the patient with a history of positive tuberculin test without active infection about environmental/occupational exposures and the type and length of the treatment, if any. The most recent appointment with the primary health provider must be recorded in the chart. Only persons with active disease are infectious to others. The medical history should include signs or symptoms of pulmonary TB, which include cough, production of sputum and blood, and chest pain. Other nonspecific symptoms, such as anorexia, fatigue, weight zon therapy. Asymptomatic individuals with a positive tuberculin test and no evidence of active pulmonary disease do not represent a risk for transmission of TB but

may be candidates for preventive therapy. Patients with a positive skin test and evidence of prior active TB by chest radiograph are also not infectious but, if not treated in the past, may also be candidates for prophylactic therapy. Patients with active disease should be on appropriate therapy. Patients should be questioned about the type of medication they are taking, the duration of the treatment, and the compliance with the regimen. Anti-tuberculosis therapy rapidly reduces the infectivity of the individual, and 2 weeks is considered adequate to label a patient as non-infectious.

Adverse reactions to TB medications may occur. The clinician should avoid medication interactions such as acetaminophen and isoniazid because of the potential for hepatotoxicity. The CDC published in 2012 "TB Elimination Infection Control in Health-Care Settings." The CDC guidelines highlight administrative controls such as delineation of policies and procedures, engineering controls such as ventilation and air flow, and personal respiratory protection.

For dental care facilities that provide care to populations at high risk of TB, engineering controls to decrease the risk of transmission should be considered. These include high efficiency ventilation and air flow (Tables 21-1 and 21-2).

Table 21-1: Dental Management of the Patient with a History of TB*		
Status	*Considerations*	*Dental Treatment*
Active sputum-positive TB	Urgent care only Consult with MD	Hospital setting with isolation If handpiece is needed (older than 6 years of age) No modification if patient is under 6 years
History of TB	Detailed medical history Obtain medical history from MD	Postpone treatment if questionable history or adequate treatment time Treat as normal patient if present status is free of clinically active disease
Recent conversion to positive skin test	Consult with MD Verify is receiving isoniazid for 6 months to 1 year for prophylaxis	Treat as normal patient
Signs or symptoms suggestive of TB	Refer to MD	Treat as active sputum positive TB

* Adapted from Little J, Falace D, Miller C, Rhodus N. Tuberculosis. *Dental Management of the Medically Compromised Patient. 7th edition.* Mosby Elsevier, 2008.

Table 21-2: Tuberculosis Precautions for Outpatient Dental Setting*	
Control	*Adjustment*
Administrative Controls	Assign responsibility for managing TB infection program Develop written TB infection control policies Instruct patient to cover mouth when coughing When hiring personnel, ensure that they are screened for latent TB infection and TB disease
Environmental Controls	Use airborne infection isolation room to provide urgent dental care treatment to patients with suspected TB
Respiratory Protection	Instruct patient to cover mouth when coughing and to wear a surgical mask Use disposable filtering face piece when providing urgent dental care to patients with suspected TB

* Adapted from Cleveland JL, Robinson VA, Panlilio AL. Tuberculosis epidemiology, diagnosis and infection control recommendations for dental setting: an update on the Centers for Disease Control and Prevention guidelines. *J Am Dent Assoc* 2009;140:1092-9.

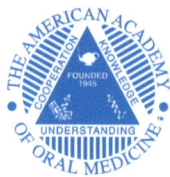

22 Legal and Ethical Issues

In June 1998, the U.S. Supreme Court ruled in Bragdon vs. Abbott, a case dealing with the Americans with Disabilities Act (AwDA). Sidney Abbott, a woman with no symptoms of HIV disclosed that she was HIV-positive when seeking dental treatment from Maine dentist, Randon Bragdon. Dr. Bragdon examined her in his dental office but refused to provide dental care in his office; instead he indicated that he would only provide care in a hospital and that Ms. Abbott would be required to bear the additional hospital expenses. Ms. Abbott brought suit under Title III of the Americans with Disabilities Act of 1990, which prohibits private providers of public accommodations (such as a private dentist) from discriminating against individuals on the basis of their disabilities.

To be protected under the AwDA, an individual must have a physical or mental impairment that substantially limits one or more major life activities, must have a record of such impairment, or be regarded as having such impairment. The AwDA permits differing treatment in cases where the individual seeking protection is not considered to be otherwise disabled, or because the individual poses a "direct threat" to himself or herself or others that cannot be eliminated through a reasonable accommodation.

The U.S. Supreme Court found HIV infection, whether symptomatic or asymptomatic, qualifies as an impairment and HIV positive individuals are protected by the AwDA, unless they pose "a direct threat to the health and safety of others. The court also found that Dr. Bragdon did not present any "objective, medical evidence" indicating that it would be safer to treat Ms. Abbott in a hospital rather than his office.

Federal law prohibits the dentist from refusing to treat patients with disabilities, including HIV. Under the Americans with Disabilities Act (AwDA), dental offices are considered places of public accommodation and are prohibited from refusing to treat HIV positive patients solely because of their HIV status. This prohibition applies not only to patients of record, but also to individuals seeking treatment for the first time. In many places, state and local laws contain comparable provisions. These laws correspond closely to the conduct required by the Principles of Ethics and Code of Professional Conduct of the American Dental Association, which specifies that patient referrals should be made whenever the welfare of patients will be safeguarded or advanced by utilizing those who have special skills, knowledge, and experience. Under the Principles, a patient's HIV status is not an appropriate basis for referral.

Under the *Health Insurance Portability and Accountability Act* (HIPAA), confidentiality of health information, including dental records, is strongly protected by law. Although HIPAA does not separately address HIV or AIDS information specifically, individuals are protected under the general guidelines regarding release of health information, including HIV status. Civil and criminal penalties can be assessed for failure to comply with mandated confidentiality regulations.

The confidentiality of dental records containing HIV-related information is specifically protected by law in most states. Although state laws vary in their strictness, a written consent from the patient for each release of HIV-related information must be obtained. State laws which are stricter than federal HIPAA regulations will take precedence. Conversely, HIPAA regulations will take precedence to less stringent state laws. The dentist is ultimately responsible for the conduct of staff and will be held responsible for any release of information.

Dentists may also be held legally liable for failing to recognize medical conditions identified while providing dental care and for failing to refer patients for follow-up care and testing. For example, recurrent oral candidiasis in a patient without a known etiology may indicate a need for referral for medical examination which may include HIV testing and counseling. Dentists are advised to be knowledgeable of their state laws regarding HIV issues and to seek the advice of legal counsel when questions arise.

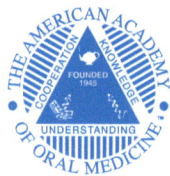

23 Infection Control Issues

Standard precautions are required for all patients because it is impossible to identify all patients with a potential to transmit infectious diseases. Many patients are asymptomatic and unaware of their infectious status, and many others may not want to tell their dental providers of their infectious status for fear of discrimination. Therefore, special infection control procedures should not be implemented for known infectious patients. A two-tier infection control program will instill a false sense of security when treating perceived noninfectious individuals and breach the confidentiality of the infectious patients.

Recent emergence of TB among the HIV positive population is of concern to dental providers, as this disease is primarily spread by airborne droplets. Elective dental procedures should be postponed until the active TB-infected patient has been cleared as noninfectious by his or her physician. At that time the patient is no longer considered contagious. A definitive non-contagious status can be confirmed by three consecutive negative sputum cultures for acid-fast bacilli. Emergency care should be provided in an appropriate negative air-pressure setting.

OCCUPATIONAL EXPOSURES AND POSTEXPOSURE PROPHYLAXIS (PEP)

It is estimated that more than 380,000 healthcare workers in the U.S annually sustain needlestick injuries. The CDC has documented of 58 documented cases of HIV seroconversion temporally associated with occupational exposure to HIV among U.S. health care personnel as of December 2013. An additional 150 cases of HIV seroconversion in healthcare workers were identified as possible sources of occupational exposure. Highest risk for occupational exposure seroconversion was associated with percutaneous injury. None of the 58 individuals were dental health care workers. In prospective studies of health care workers in hospital settings, the average risk of HIV transmission after a percutaneous exposure to HIV-infected blood has been estimated to be approximately 0.3% (3 out of 1,000) and after mucous membrane exposure, approximately 0.09% (<1 out of 1,000). HIV seroconversion rates are exceedingly small when compared to seroconversion rates for HBV (23-37% for HBsAg$^+$ and HBeAg$^-$ and 37–62% for HBsAg$^-$ and HBeAg$^+$ source patient blood) and lower than HCV (1.8% average, 0–7% range).

In September 2013, the U.S. Public Health Service published the Updated U.S. Public Health Service Guidelines for the Management of Occupational Exposures to HIV and Recommendations for Postexposure Prophylaxis. These guidelines contain recommendations for the management of health care personnel occupational exposures to blood and other body fluids that might contain HIV. These guideline update previously published guidelines. These 2013 guidelines modify and expand the list of antiretroviral medications that can be considered for use as post exposure prophylaxis (PEP). This report also emphasizes prompt management of occupational exposures, selection of tolerable regimens, attention to potential drug interactions involving drugs that could be included in HIV PEP regimens and other medications, consultation with experts for post-exposure management strategies and selection of HIV PEP regimens, use of HIV rapid testing, and counseling and follow-up of exposed personnel. Guidelines for exposure to HBV and HCV have been published previously and are not included in the 2013 report.

All health care facilities should have a written blood borne pathogen policy that includes management of exposures.

The U.S. Public Health Service no longer recommends the severity of exposure to determine the number of drugs to be offered in an HIV PEP regimen. When a healthcare provider has been exposed to a source person who has HIV infection or for whom there is reasonable suspicion of HIV infection PEP should be offered. When PEP is offered and taken and the source is later determined to be HIV negative, PEP should be discontinued, and no further HIV follow-up testing is indicated for the exposed provider. Since most all occupational HIV exposures do not result in transmission of HIV, the risks of PEP including the potential for severe toxicity and drug interactions must be considered carefully when prescribing PEP. A regimen containing 3 (or more) antiretroviral drugs is now recommended routinely for all occupational exposures to HIV. Examples of recom-

TABLE 23-1: MANAGEMENT OF OCCUPATIONAL BLOOD EXPOSURES TO HIV	
Provide immediate care to the exposure site.	Wash wounds and skin with soap and water. Flush mucous membranes with water.
Reporting of exposure.	Access to medical provider for testing. Access to post-exposure protocol. Documentation for workers compensation or disability claims.
Determine risk associated with exposure by:	Type of fluid (e.g., blood, visibly bloody fluid, other potentially infectious fluid or tissue, and concentrated virus) and Type of exposure (i.e., percutaneous injury, mucous membrane or non intact skin exposure, and bites resulting in blood exposure).
Evaluate exposure source.	Assess the risk of infection using available information. Test known sources for HBsAg, anti-HCV, and HIV antibody (consider using rapid testing). For unknown sources, assess risk of exposure to HBV, HCV, or HIV infection. Do not test discarded needles or syringes for virus contamination.
Evaluate exposed person	Assess immune status for HBV infection (i.e., by history of HBV vaccination and vaccine response).
Give PEP for exposures posing risk of infection transmission.	HBV – If source patient HBsAg+ or unknown, check HBsAb status of exposed. If exposed is unvaccinated or non responder (<10 mIU/mL): HBIGx1 and initiate HB vaccination HCV – PEP not recommended HIV – PEP recommendations if source patient is HIV seropositive or is reasonable assumed to be HIV seropositive. Initiate PEP as soon as possible, preferably within hours of exposure. Offer pregnancy testing to all women of childbearing age not known to be pregnant. Seek expert consultation if viral resistance is suspected Administer PEP for 4 weeks if tolerated.
Perform follow-up testing and provide counseling.	Advise exposed persons to seek medical evaluation for any acute illness occurring during follow-up. Discontinue PEP if source patient is subsequently HIV seronegative.
HBV exposures	Perform follow-up anti-HBs testing in persons who receive HB vaccine. Test for anti-HBs 1-2 months after last dose of vaccine. Anti-HBs response to vaccine cannot be ascertained if HBIG was received in the previous 3-4 months.
HCV exposures	Perform baseline and follow-up testing for anti-HCV and alanine amino-transferase (ALT) 4-6 months after exposure. Perform HCV RNA at 4-6 weeks if earlier diagnosis of HCV infection is desired. Confirm repeatedly reactive anti-HCV enzyme immunoassays (EIAs) with supplemental tests.
HIV exposures	Perform HIV antibody testing by enzyme immunoassay for at least 6 months post-exposure (e.g., at baseline, 6 weeks, 3 months, and 6 months). Perform HIV antibody testing if illness compatible with an acute retroviral syndrome occurs. Advise exposed person to use precautions, such as barrier contraception or abstinence to prevent secondary transmission during the follow-up period. Evaluate exposed person taking PEP within 72 hours after exposure to monitor for drug toxicity for at least 2 weeks.

mended PEP regimens include those consisting of a dual nucleoside reverse transcriptase inhibitors (NRTIs) plus an integrase strand transfer inhibitors (INSTIs), a protease inhibitor (PI), or a non nucleoside reverse transcriptase inhibitor (NNRTI). Other antiretroviral drug combinations may be indicated for specific cases (e.g., exposure to a source patient harboring drug-resistant HIV) but should be prescribed only after consultation with an expert in the use of antiretroviral agents.

Staff Training

To reduce fear and apprehension when treating known HIV positive patients it is critical that all dental personnel be properly trained in HIV disease pathogenesis and transmission. Moreover, epidemiology, oral and systemic manifestations, legal and ethical issues, and psychosocial considerations training should also be included. Frequent information and training sessions need to be instituted in which up-to-date information can be discussed. These sessions should also address concerns and issues that have arisen during the treatment of HIV positive patients.

Psychosocial Considerations

The dental healthcare team is faced with two major psychosocial issues when treating HIV positive patients: the psychosocial effect of the disease on the patients and the psychosocial effect of the disease on the healthcare providers.

Patients may experience periods of denial, fear, anger, disbelief, guilt and anxiety about death during the progression of their disease, which can directly influence the patient-dentist relationship. Patients' concerns about transmitting HIV to healthcare providers may even determine the treatment they are prepared to undergo.

For healthcare providers it is important to recognize and acknowledge their fears of HIV transmission and contagion, as well as pressure from peer groups and family members to avoid treating HIV positive patients. Social stigmas associated with this disease can also be affixed to the healthcare worker who treats a large number of HIV positive patients, who may erroneously be perceived as having the virus or as being a member of an HIV risk group. Another difficult issue for the dental team is treating young patients diagnosed with a potentially fatal disease. Dentists who have traditionally been trained in treating healthy ambulatory patients are faced with incorporating severely medically complex patients into a general dental office setting.

To better cope with these issues it may be necessary to provide psychological support mechanisms for dental providers, especially those who deal with large numbers of AIDS patients.

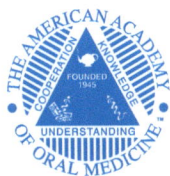

Appendix – AIDS Defining Conditions

AIDS DEFINING CONDITIONS FOR ADOLESCENTS AND ADULTS

- Bacterial infections, multiple or recurrent *
- Candidiasis of bronchi, trachea, or lungs
- Candidiasis of esophagus †
- Cervical cancer, invasive §
- Coccidioidomycosis, disseminated or extrapulmonary
- Cryptococcosis, extrapulmonary
- Cryptosporidiosis, chronic intestinal (>1 month's duration)
- Cytomegalovirus disease (other than liver, spleen, or nodes), onset at age >1 month
- Cytomegalovirus retinitis (with loss of vision) †
- Encephalopathy, HIV related
- Herpes simplex: chronic ulcers (>1 month's duration) or bronchitis, pneumonitis, or esophagitis (onset at age >1 month)
- Histoplasmosis, disseminated or extrapulmonary
- Isosporiasis, chronic intestinal (>1 month's duration)
- Kaposi sarcoma †
- Lymphoid interstitial pneumonia or pulmonary lymphoid hyperplasia complex *†
- Lymphoma, Burkitt (or equivalent term)
- Lymphoma, immunoblastic (or equivalent term)
- Lymphoma, primary, of brain
- Mycobacterium avium complex or Mycobacterium kansasii, disseminated or extrapulmonary †
- Mycobacterium tuberculosis of any site, pulmonary,†§ disseminated,† or extrapulmonary †
- Mycobacterium, other species or unidentified species, disseminated† or extrapulmonary †
- Pneumocystis jirovecii pneumonia †
- Pneumonia, recurrent †§
- Progressive multifocal leukoencephalopathy
- Salmonella septicemia, recurrent
- Toxoplasmosis of brain, onset at age >1 month †
- Wasting syndrome attributed to HIV

* Only among children aged <13 years. (*Centers for Disease Control and Prevention. 1994 Revised classification system for human immunodeficiency virus infection in children less than 13 years of age. MMWR 1994;43[No. RR-12].*)
† Condition that might be diagnosed presumptively.
§ Only among adults and adolescents aged >13 years.

Centers for Disease Control and Prevention. 1993 Revised classification system for HIV infection and expanded surveillance case definition for AIDS among adolescents and adults. MMWR 1992;41(No. RR-17).

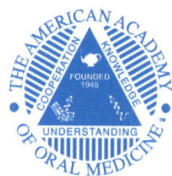

Patient Material/Resources

INTERNET RESOURCES	
Organizations & Commercial sites:	
HIVDENT	http://www.hivdent.org/
The Body	http://www.thebody.com/
Project Inform	http://www.projectinform.org/
American Foundation for AIDS Research	http://www.amfar.org/
New York State Department of Health AIDS Institute Resources	http://www.hivguidelines.org/
AIDS Clinical Trials Group Network	https://actgnetwork.org/
CDC National Prevention Information Network	http://www.cdcnpin.org
US Government sites:	
Health Resources & Services Administration (HRSA) HIV/AIDS Programs	http://hab.hrsa.gov/
National Institutes of Health (NIH)	http://www.nih.gov/
National Institute of Allergy and Infectious Disease (NIAID)	http://www.niaid.nih.gov/
Centers for Disease Control and Prevention (CDC)	http://www.cdc.gov/default.htm
CDC Division of HIV/AIDS Prevention	https://www.cdc.gov/hiv/library/factsheets/index.html
International sites:	
World Health Organization (WHO)	http://www.who.int/en
UNAIDS	http://unaidstoday.org/

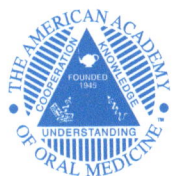

Additional Readings

- Abubakar I., M. Lipman, T.D. McHugh, H. Fletcher. 2016. Uniting to end the TB epidemic: Advances in disease control from prevention to better diagnosis and treatment. *BMC Medicine*. 14 doi:http://dx.doi.org/10.1186/s12916-016-0599-1

- Beachler D.C., K.M. Weber, J.B. Margolick, et al. 2012. Risk Factors for Oral HPV Infection among a High Prevalence Population of HIV-Positive and At-Risk HIV-Negative Adults.Cancer *Epidemiol Biomarkers Prev*. (21)(1):122-133.

- Filteau S., G. PrayGod, L. Kasonka, et al. 2015. Effects on mortality of a nutritional intervention for malnourished HIV-infected adults referred for antiretroviral therapy: a randomised controlled trial. *BMC Med*. 13:17

- Kim A. 2016. Hepatitis C Virus. *Annals of Internal Medicine* 165(5):ITC33-ITC48.

- Kuhar D.T., D.K. Henderson, K.A. Struble, W. Heneine, V. Thomas, L.W. Cheever, A. Gomaa, A.L. Panlilio, US Public Health Service Working Group. 2013. Updated US Public Health Service guidelines for the management of occupational exposures to human immunodeficiency virus and recommendations for postexposure prophylaxis. *Infect Control Hosp Epidemiol*. Sep 34(9):875-92.

- Patton L.L. 2016. Current strategies for prevention of oral manifestations of human immunodeficiency virus. *Oral Surg Oral Med Oral Pathol Oral Radiol*. 121:29-38

- Robbins M.R. 2017. Recent Recommendations for Management of Human Immunodeficiency Virus–Positive Patients. *Dental Clinics of North America* 61:365-387

- Scott L., P. da Silva, C.C. Boehme, W. Stevens, C. Gilpin. 2017. Diagnosis of opportunistic infections: HIV co-infections–tuberculosis. *Curr Opin HIV AIDS* 12:129–138. (RR-10):1-12.

- Selik R.M., E.D. Mokotoff, B. Branson, et al. 2014. Centers for Disease Control and Prevention (CDC) Revised surveillance case definition for HIV infection–United States, *MMWR Recomm. Rep.*, 63 (RR-03), pp. 1-10

- Shiboski C.H., L.L. Patton, J.Y. Webster-Cyriaque, D. Greenspan, R.S. Traboulsi, M. Ghannoum, et al. 2009. The Oral HIV/AIDS Research Alliance: updated case definitions of oral disease endpoints. *J Oral Pathol Med*. 38:481–488.

- Shiboski C.H., J.Y. Webster-Cyriaque, M. Ghannoum, et al. 2016. The Oral HIV/AIDS Research Alliance Program: lessons learned and future directions. *Oral Dis*. 22(S1):128-134

- Tang A.M., T. Quick, M. Chung, et al. 2015. Nutrition assessment, counseling, and support interventions to Improve Health-Related outcomes in people living with HIV/AIDS: a systematic review of the literature. *J Acquir Immune Defic Syndr*. 68 (suppl 3):S340–S349.

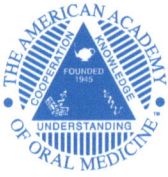

The American Academy of Oral Medicine
2150 N. 107th St., Suite 205
Seattle, Washington 98133
PHONE: (206) 209-5279 · EMAIL: info@aaom.com

Application for AAOM Membership

ELIGIBILITY FOR MEMBERSHIP

1. Nominee for **Regular Membership** shall be a graduate of an accredited Dental School or Medicine School and shall be a member of his/her representative National Society and shall pursue special interest or accomplishment in the field of Oral Medicine.

2. Nominee for **Affiliate Membership** (student) shall be a graduate of an accredited Dental or Medical School and shall be a member of his/her representative National Society and currently in training in a Postdoctoral program.

3. Nominee for **Student Membership** shall be a student currently enrolled in a pre-doctoral program in an accredited dental or medical school. Students are those seeking a DDS, DMD or MD degree.

4. The fiscal year for dues starts January 1.

5. After acceptance into the Academy, Active Membership dues are paid annually and include a subscription to ORAL SURGERY, ORAL MEDICINE, ORAL PATHOLOGY, ORAL RADIOLOGY, and ENDODONTOLOGY.

6. Please see the AAOM website for more membership information and how to apply: www.aaom.com.

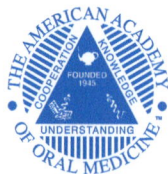